RENAL DIET COOKBOOK

FOR BEGINNERS

The Unique Year-Round Kidney Health Cookbook, Start Anytime with Easy, Delicious Recipes for Managing Kidney Disease – Low in Sodium, Potassium, and Phosphorus, Plus Expert Tips and Nutrition Insights for a Healthier You

By Joyna E. Dwait

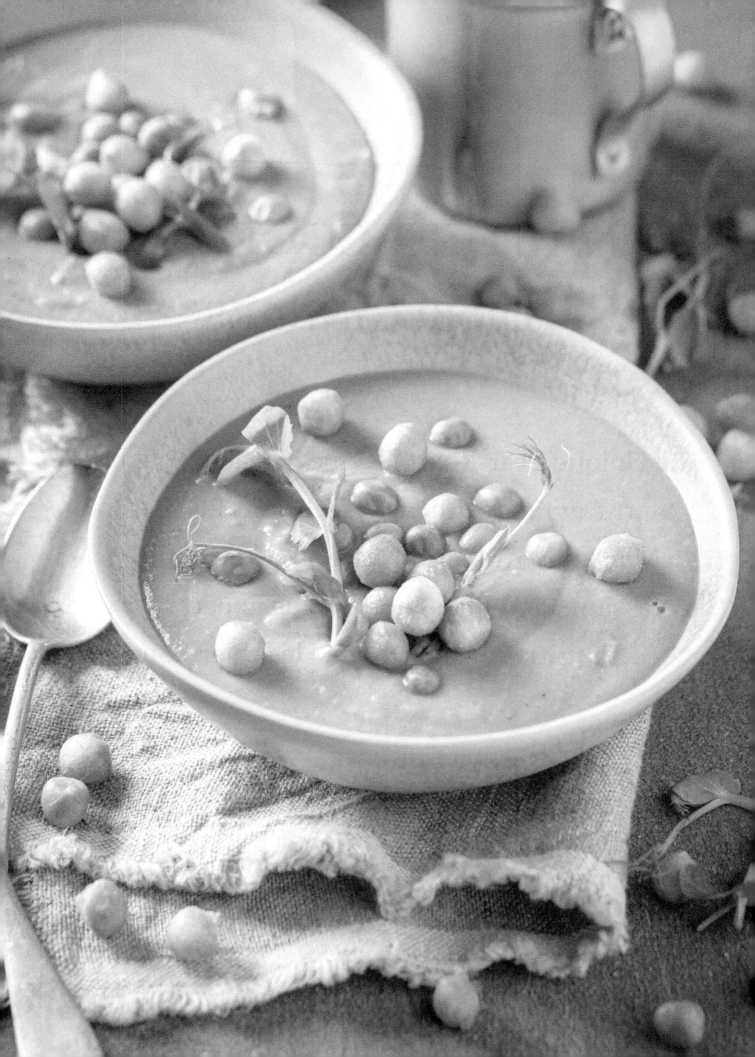

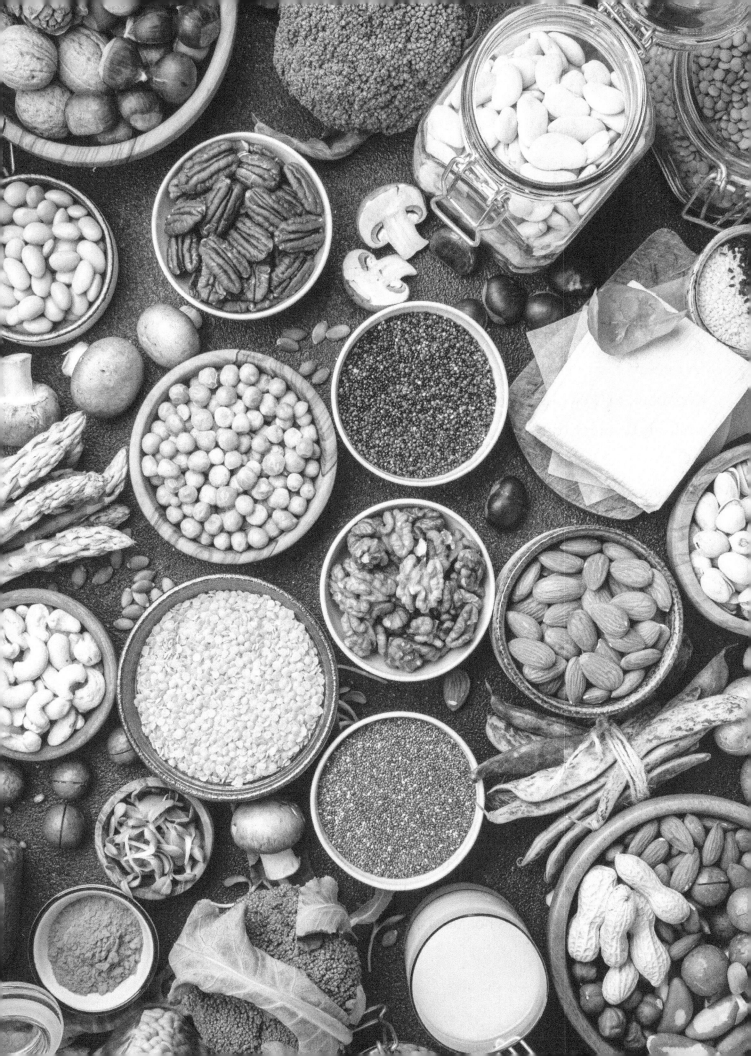

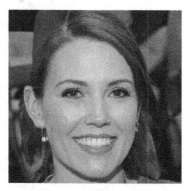

Joyna E. Dwait, an impassioned culinary artist and a beacon of hope for those embarking on a renal health journey, authors the transformative "Renal Diet Cookbook for Beginners." With a heart as nourishing as her recipes, Joyna has become synonymous with a life of flavor and health. Her journey, fueled by a profound commitment to well-being and an innate love for the culinary arts, has led to a book that's more than just a collection of recipes—it's an invitation to a healthier, more vibrant life. Joyna's warmth and wisdom leap off every page, guiding readers with care and inspiring a new chapter in their dietary lives.

"A Lifesaver in Every Sense" Joyna's book has been a godsend for our family. The 'Renal Diet Cookbook for Beginners' isn't just a set of recipes; it's a new lease on life. Every dish brings a smile and health to our table. It's a must-have for anyone on a renal diet.

"Deliciously Healing" Never knew a diet book could be so delightful! Joyna's creations are easy, tasty, and above all, healing. My kitchen has never seen so much joy and health. This book is a treasure for anyone facing renal health challenges.

"Transformative & Tasty!" Joyna E. Dwait turns dietary restrictions into a culinary celebration. Each recipe in her 'Renal Diet Cookbook for Beginners' is a step toward better health without ever missing a beat on flavor. I'm truly grateful for this book!

"Heartfelt and Healthy" Joyna's approach to the renal diet is a heartfelt blend of taste and health. Her book has not just changed my diet; it's changed my outlook on life. It's a must-read for those on a health journey.

"Culinary Genius for Health" Each page of 'Renal Diet Cookbook for Beginners' is a brushstroke in Joyna's masterpiece of healthful eating. The recipes are approachable, delicious, and incredibly beneficial. It's not just a cookbook; it's a path to wellness."

Hello, wonderful reader!

I hope you'll enjoy embarking on the path to kidney health and delightful flavors with "Renal Diet Cookbook for Beginners"!

To enjoy the **extra care** your diet deserves,
just scan the **QR code** here and discover more enriching recipes and insightful tips:

Thank you
for choosing this taste bud friendly book! #FlavorfulWellness

TABLE OF CONTENT

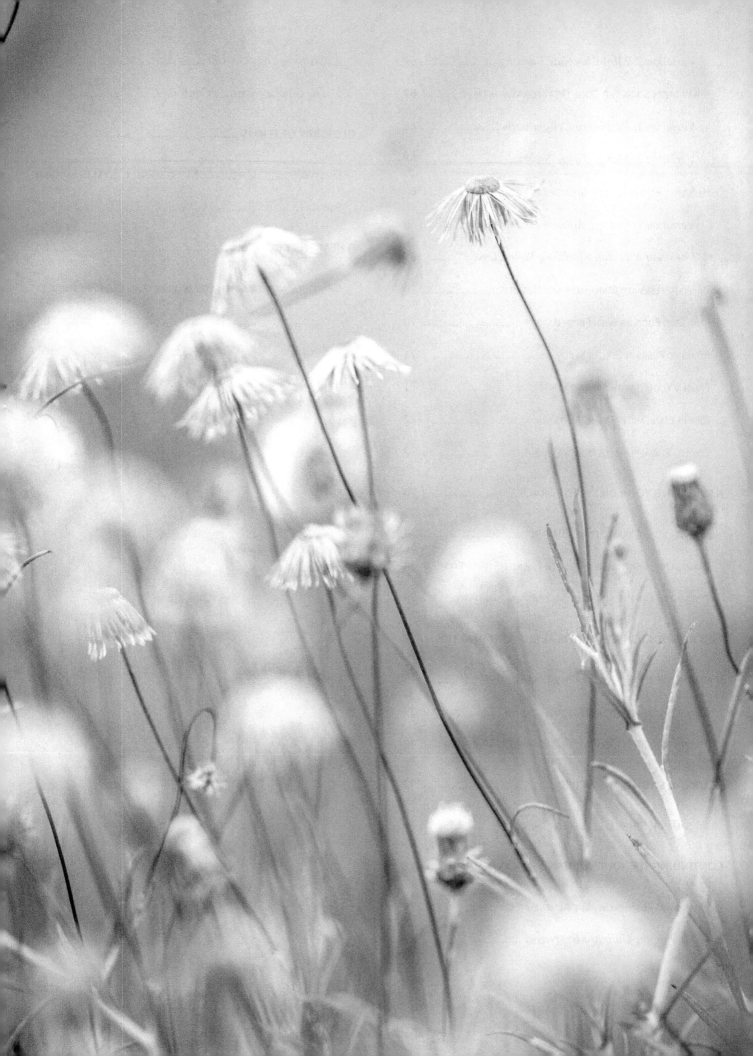

Embarking on Your Culinary Adventure with a Trusted Friend!

Welcome to a culinary adventure that's not just about food, but also about nourishing your body and soul. Whether you're embarking on this journey to support a loved one or are personally navigating the intricate landscape of a renal diet, you're not alone. Together, we'll discover the profound impact that mindful eating can have on our well-being and how simple, yet innovative culinary choices can make a significant difference in our health. Food is more than mere sustenance; it is a source of comfort, joy, and connection. Sharing a meal with a loved one, experimenting with new flavors, and savoring every bite can be deeply fulfilling. However, the path to culinary satisfaction can feel challenging when health concerns call for a strict dietary regimen. This cookbook aims to transform that challenge into an opportunity—an opportunity to explore, create, and relish delicious meals while honoring the guidelines of a renal diet.

A Warm Welcome: Embracing the Journey Together

Embarking on a culinary adventure can be an exciting and rewarding experience, but it can also be a daunting one, especially if you're dealing with specific dietary restrictions. In this journey, we'll not only be your trusted friend but also your guide through the world of the renal diet. Whether you or a loved one are facing kidney health challenges, it's important to understand that the right diet can make a significant difference in your overall well-being.

At times, navigating a renal diet can seem like a lonely path, filled with restrictions and uncertainties. That's why we're here to emphasize the "together" in this culinary adventure. By sharing knowledge, tips, and recipes, we hope to create this journey more enjoyable, manageable, and, most importantly, fulfilling. Remember, you're not alone, and there's a community of individuals just like you, embracing the renal diet to live a healthier life.

The renal diet is a specialized dietary plan designed to support kidney function and manage kidney-related health issues. It's not just about what you can't eat; it's about what you can eat and relish while still taking care of your health. You'll discover that the key to success is not only in understanding the restrictions but in creatively incorporating the right components and flavors into your meals.

As we embark on this culinary adventure, let's set the stage for what's to come. Imagine your kitchen as a portal to better health, and each recipe as a step forward on the path to nourishing your body and your spirit. Together, we'll explore a world of delicious and kidney-friendly dishes that will leave you feeling satisfied and well-cared for.

The heart of this journey is understanding the renal diet's core principles and transforming that knowledge into nourishing meals that you and your loved ones will cherish. So, let's dive into the fundamental aspects of the renal diet, which is the key to embracing this adventure together.

The Heart of the Renal Diet: Turning Knowledge into Nourishment

The renal diet is designed to minimize the strain on your kidneys by managing the intake of certain nutrients like sodium, potassium, phosphorus, and protein. This, in turn, helps prevent complications associated with kidney disease, such as fluid retention, high blood pressure, and mineral imbalances.

As we embrace the principles of the renal diet, it's important to remember that it's not about deprivation or bland meals. Instead, it's an opportunity to get creative in the kitchen and explore a world of flavors and textures that align with your health goals.

In this cookbook, you'll find a diverse range of recipes, carefully crafted to adhere to the renal diet's principles. These recipes offer a delightful fusion of components, techniques, and flavors that transform every meal into a culinary adventure.

Every recipe in this cookbook has been designed with your renal health in mind, while not compromising on taste. We'll provide clear instructions and essential nutritional information for each dish, making it easy to plan your meals and manage your dietary restrictions.

So, dear reader, get ready to embark on a culinary journey that balances knowledge and nourishment. With our trusted guidance, you'll not only embrace the renal diet but also savor every bite of this delectable adventure. Let's get started!

Laying the Foundations with Care

Before we embark on this culinary adventure, it's crucial to have a reliable compass guiding our way—the understanding of the renal diet. Knowledge is power, and in this case, it's the power to maintain your kidney health while relishing the flavors of your meals.

The Compass: Understanding the Renal Diet

The renal diet, also known as the kidney diet, is a specialized dietary plan designed to support individuals with kidney disease. Kidneys play a vital role in filtering waste and extra fluids from the blood, regulating electrolyte balance, and maintaining overall homeostasis in the body. When kidney function is impaired, it becomes necessary to adjust one's diet to reduce the workload on the kidneys and manage various health complications associated with kidney disease. This comprehensive guide will delve into the fundamentals of the renal diet, including its purpose, key components, recommended food choices, dietary restrictions, and practical tips for maintaining a healthy & balanced lifestyle while managing kidney disease.

Purpose of the Renal Diet

The primary purpose of the renal diet is to reduce the strain on the kidneys by limiting the intake of substances that can be harmful when not effectively filtered by these vital organs. It aims to:

1. **Manage Fluid Balance:** One of the key functions of the kidneys is to regulate fluid balance in the body. In kidney disease, this balance is disrupted, leading to fluid retention, swelling (edema), and increased blood pressure. The renal diet helps control fluid intake to prevent these issues.

2. **Minimize Toxin Accumulation:** Healthy kidneys filter waste and toxins from the bloodstream. When kidney function is impaired, these substances can build up in the body, leading to a condition known as uremia. The renal diet reduces the intake of substances that can contribute to this buildup.

3. **Regulate Electrolyte Levels:** Kidneys help maintain the balance of essential electrolytes, such as potassium, sodium, and phosphorus, in the body. Kidney disease can disrupt this balance, and the renal diet is designed to manage these electrolyte levels.

4. **Prevent Protein Breakdown:** As the kidneys lose function, the body's ability to eliminate waste products from protein metabolism decreases. By controlling protein intake, the renal diet helps minimize the accumulation of waste products, particularly urea.

Key Components of the Renal Diet

The renal diet is characterized by several key components, each of which serves a specific purpose in managing kidney disease:

1. **Fluid Control:** People with kidney disease are often advised to limit their fluid intake. This restriction helps prevent fluid retention, swelling, and high blood pressure. It's crucial to monitor and limit the consumption of beverages like water, juice, and soda, as well as foods with high water content, such as watermelon and cucumber.

2. **Protein Restriction:** Reducing protein intake is a fundamental aspect of the renal diet. Protein metabolism produces waste products like urea, which the kidneys have difficulty eliminating when impaired. Limiting protein helps prevent the buildup of these waste products. However, it's important to consume enough high-quality protein to maintain overall health and prevent malnutrition.

3. **Sodium Control:** Excessive sodium (salt) intake can lead to fluid retention and high blood pressure, which are detrimental to kidney health. The renal diet emphasizes limiting sodium intake by avoiding high-salt foods like processed and fast foods.

4. **Potassium Management:** Proper potassium levels are crucial for maintaining heart and muscle function. Kidney disease can lead to abnormal potassium levels, potentially causing heart rhythm problems. The renal diet includes recommendations to control potassium intake by avoiding high-potassium foods like bananas, oranges, and potatoes.

5. **Phosphorus Regulation:** The kidneys are responsible for removing extra phosphorus from the blood. In kidney disease, this regulation is impaired, leading to high phosphorus levels, which can weaken bones and damage blood vessels. The renal diet involves limiting phosphorus intake by avoiding foods rich in phosphorus, such as dairy products and certain beans.

6. **Adequate Calories:** Despite the restrictions on protein, sodium, potassium, and phosphorus, it's essential for individuals with kidney disease to maintain an adequate calorie intake. This ensures they have enough energy to support their daily activities and prevent malnutrition.

Recommended Food Choices

The renal diet emphasizes specific food choices to help individuals with kidney disease manage their condition effectively. Here are some recommendations for each key component of the renal diet:

Fluid Control

• Limit water and other fluids as recommended by your healthcare provider.

• Monitor your daily fluid intake to avoid exceeding your prescribed limit.

• Choose ice chips or small sips of water to moisten your mouth instead of drinking big amounts at once.

• Be mindful of foods with high water content, like soups, gelatin, and ice cream.

Protein Restriction

- Choose high-quality protein sources, such as poultry, lean meat, fish, and eggs.
- Limit your portion sizes of protein-rich foods.
- Use plant-based protein sources, such as tofu and legumes, as they generally have lower protein content than animal sources.
- Consider working with a registered dietitian to calculate and customize your daily protein allowance based on your individual needs.

Sodium Control

- Avoid high-sodium foods, including processed, tinned, and fast foods.
- Use herbs and spices to flavour your food instead of salt.
- Read food labels to identify hidden sources of sodium in packaged products.
- Choose fresh, whole foods and cook at home to have better control over your sodium intake.

Potassium Management

- Limit or avoid high-potassium fruits and vegetables like bananas, oranges, and potatoes.
- Opt for lower-potassium alternatives, such as apples, berries, and green beans.
- Cooking methods, like leaching or soaking, can reduce the potassium content in certain foods.
- Consult with a dietitian to create a personalized potassium management plan.

Phosphorus Regulation

- Limit dairy products, including milk, cheese, and yogurt, as they are rich in phosphorus.
- Choose phosphorus binders as prescribed by your healthcare provider to help control phosphorus absorption.
- Be cautious with processed and fast foods, as they often contain additives and preservatives high in phosphorus.
- Include white bread, rice, and pasta in your diet, as they generally have lower phosphorus content than whole grains.

Adequate Calories

- Focus on calorie-dense foods like healthy fats (avocado, nuts, and olive oil) and complex carbohydrates (whole grains, legumes, and vegetables).
- Work with a dietitian to create a meal plan that ensures you meet your calorie needs while adhering to other dietary restrictions.

Dietary Restrictions

While the renal diet provides guidelines for managing kidney disease, it also involves certain dietary restrictions to protect the kidneys and overall health. Understanding and adhering to these restrictions is essential for effective management of kidney disease:

1. **Avoid High-Sodium Foods:** High-sodium foods, such as processed meats, tinned soups, and fast food, can contribute to fluid retention and elevated blood pressure. Reducing sodium intake is crucial for kidney health.

2. **Limit High-Potassium Foods:** Foods like bananas, oranges, and potatoes are rich in potassium, and individuals with kidney disease should limit their consumption to prevent high potassium levels, which can be dangerous for the heart.

3. **Minimize High-Phosphorus Foods:** Dairy products, certain legumes, and processed foods often contain high levels of phosphorus. Reducing phosphorus intake helps protect bone health and maintain cardiovascular health.

4. **Control Fluid Intake:** Staying within the prescribed fluid limits is essential to manage fluid retention, swelling, and hypertension, which are common complications of kidney disease.

5. **Monitor Protein Intake:** While it's important to consume enough protein to prevent malnutrition, excessive protein intake can strain the kidneys. Work with a healthcare provider or dietitian to determine your individual protein needs.

6. **Limit High-Purine Foods:** High-purine foods, such as organ meats, shellfish, and certain fish, can lead to the accumulation of uric acid in the body, potentially exacerbating kidney disease.

Nutrients: Your Trusty Travel Companions

Now that you understand the renal diet's fundamentals, let's get to know your trusty travel companions—nutrients. Your journey towards better kidney health will be guided by the right balance of nutrients, each playing a unique role in your dietary plan.

1. **Fiber:** A renal diet should not exclude fiber. It helps in managing blood sugar levels and maintains digestive health. Incorporate whole grains, fruits, and vegetables in your meals to ensure an adequate fiber intake.

2. **Calcium:** Maintaining healthy bones is essential, especially for individuals with kidney issues. While high-phosphorus dairy products are restricted, you can still get your calcium from low-phosphorus options like almond milk or fortified cereals.

3. **Iron:** Some renal patients may experience anemia, which is why iron intake is important. Lean cuts of meat, poultry, and fish are excellent sources of iron. Pair them with foods rich in vitamin C to enhance iron absorption.

16

4. **Vitamin D:** Proper kidney function is required for the activation of vitamin D in the body. If your kidneys are compromised, your healthcare provider may recommend supplements to ensure you get enough vitamin D.

5. **B Vitamins:** B vitamins play a crucial role in various bodily functions, including energy metabolism. Whole grains, lean meats, and eggs are great sources of B vitamins.

6. **Antioxidants:** Antioxidants help combat free radicals, reducing oxidative stress. Incorporate colorful fruits and vegetables in your diet for a wide range of antioxidants.

Understanding the role of these nutrients will help you make informed choices when selecting components for your meals. Keep in mind that a balanced diet, even with dietary restrictions, can provide the nutrients your body needs to stay strong and healthy.

Quenching Thirst: Crafting Beverages with Love

Staying hydrated is important, but it can be a bit more complicated on a renal diet. You'll need to pay close attention to your fluid intake, as overconsumption can lead to swelling and high blood pressure. Crafting beverages that quench your thirst while adhering to the renal diet principles is not only doable but also enjoyable.

Fluid Intake Management

Understanding the source of your fluid intake is key. Besides the fluids you drink, you should also consider the fluid content of certain foods. Water, ice cubes, and watery fruits and vegetables like watermelon and cucumbers all count towards your daily fluid intake.

Kidney-Friendly Beverage Options

1. **Water:** The ultimate hydrator. Keep a reusable water bottle with you throughout the day to track your intake.

2. **Herbal Teas:** Many herbal teas are caffeine-free and can be a pleasant way to stay hydrated. Look for options like chamomile, hibiscus, or mint.

3. **Fruit-Infused Water:** Include a splash of natural flavor to your water by infusing it with slices of citrus fruits, berries, or cucumber.

4. **Homemade Lemonade:** Make a kidney-friendly lemonade using fresh lemon juice, water, and a touch of sugar or a sugar substitute.

5. **Homemade Smoothies:** Create delicious smoothies using low-potassium fruits, like berries and apples, along with non-dairy milk and ice.

6. **Diluted Fruit Juices:** You can relish a small serving of diluted fruit juice to include a burst of flavor to your beverages.

Beverage No-No's

1. **Sodas:** Regular and diet sodas are generally high in phosphorus and should be avoided.

2. **Caffeinated Beverages:** Caffeine can lead to dehydration, so it's best to limit or avoid caffeinated drinks like coffee and black tea.

3. **Alcohol:** Alcohol can be dehydrating and may interact with medications, so it's wise to consult your healthcare provider regarding alcohol consumption.

By carefully selecting and crafting your beverages, you can maintain proper hydration without putting excessive strain on your kidneys. Remember to monitor your fluid intake as advised by your healthcare provider to ensure it aligns with your specific needs.

Setting Up Your Cozy Kitchen Sanctuary

Creating a warm and inviting kitchen sanctuary is an essential step in your culinary adventure. Here, we'll guide you through the process of setting up your kitchen with the right tools, stocking your pantry with care and thought, and mastering the art of smart shopping. With the right foundation, your culinary journey will be even more enjoyable and efficient.

Essential Tools: Your Reliable Kitchen Allies

A well-equipped kitchen is the cornerstone of any successful culinary adventure. Your kitchen tools are like trusted allies, ready to assist you in crafting delicious and nourishing meals while adhering to the renal diet. Let's explore the essential tools that will make your cooking journey more enjoyable and efficient.

1. **Cutting Boards:** Invest in good quality cutting boards, preferably separate ones for fruits and vegetables and another for meats. This minimizes the risk of cross-contamination.

2. **Knives:** A set of sharp, high-quality knives is essential. Look for a paring knife, chef's knife, and serrated knife to cover all your cutting needs.

3. **Pots & Pans**: A variety of pots and pans in different sizes will present you well. A non-stick frying pan, a saucepan, a stockpot, and a sauté pan are good basics to have.

4. **Blender or Food Processor:** These appliances are excellent for creating smooth purees, soups, and kidney-friendly smoothies.

5. **Measuring Cups and Spoons:** Precise measurements are crucial in cooking. Make sure to have a set of measuring teacups and spoons to ensure your recipes come out as intended.

6. **Mixing Bowls:** A selection of mixing containers in various sizes will be invaluable for preparing components and mixing dishes.

7. **Colander:** For rinsing fruits, vegetables, and draining pasta.

8. **Baking Sheets and Pans:** If you relish baking, make sure you have a selection of baking sheets and pans for sweet treats or savory dishes.

9. **Utensils:** Stock up on spatulas, tongs, whisks, and ladles to create cooking and serving a breeze.

10. **Thermometer:** A food thermometer ensures that meats and poultry are cooked to the right internal temp., promoting both safety and taste.

11. **Can Opener:** Choose a sturdy can opener for easy access to tinned components, like low-sodium beans and vegetables.

12. **Garlic Press:** If you use garlic frequently, a press can save you time and effort.

13. **Grater and Zester:** For adding flavor with grated citrus zest or cheese.

14. **Oven Mitts:** Protect your hands when handling hot dishes and cookware.

15. **Storage Containers:** Invest in a variety of airtight containers for storing leftovers and prepared components.

The Heartfelt Pantry: Stocking Up with Care and Thought

A well-stocked pantry is the backbone of efficient cooking. It ensures you have the basics on hand to whip up meals without the need for constant trips to the grocery store. Here's a list of pantry staples for your renal diet kitchen.

1. **Low-Sodium Broth:** This is a versatile ingredient for soups and stews. Look for low-sodium or no-salt-added options.

2. **Canned Low-Potassium Vegetables:** Choose options like green beans, wax beans, or carrots.

3. **Canned Low-Potassium Fruits:** Opt for fruits like peaches, pears, or pineapple.

4. **Canned Beans:** Go for low-sodium or no-salt-added tinned beans. They're a great source of plant-based protein.

5. **Rice and Pasta:** Keep a variety of renal-friendly grains on hand, such as white rice, pasta, and couscous.

6. **Low-Sodium Condiments:** Stock up on low-sodium soy sauce, low-sodium ketchup, and salt-free herb and spice blends.

7. **Cooking Oils:** Choose kidney-friendly oils like olive oil, canola oil, or grapeseed oil.

8. **Flour Alternatives:** If you're into baking, explore kidney-friendly flour alternatives like almond flour or coconut flour.

9. **Low-Phosphorus Cereals:** Look for cereals that are low in phosphorus and low in potassium to start your day with a kidney-friendly breakfast.

10. **Dried Herbs and Spices:** Build a collection of dried herbs and spices to include flavor to your dishes without relying on salt.

11. **Low-Phosphorus Snacks:** Explore snacks like rice cakes, popcorn, or low-phosphorus crackers for those in-between meal munchies.

12. **Nuts and Seeds:** Keep kidney-friendly nuts and seeds like almonds, cashews, and chia seeds for added texture and flavor.

13. **Vinegar:** Stock up on vinegar options like balsamic vinegar or rice vinegar to include a tangy punch to your meals.

14. **Sugar Alternatives:** Choose kidney-friendly sugar substitutes like stevia or erythritol.

By keeping these pantry staples on hand, you'll always have the foundation for a variety of renal diet-friendly dishes. It makes meal preparation more convenient and helps you maintain a diet that's both healthy and delicious.

Smart Shopping: Decoding Food Labels with Ease

Navigating the grocery store with a renal diet in mind can be a breeze with a little knowledge about how to read food labels. Let's break down the essential tips for smart shopping.

15. **Sodium Content:** Look for products labeled as "low-sodium" or "no salt added." Compare the sodium content on the Nutrition Facts label to choose the lowest option.

16. **Potassium Content:** Unfortunately, potassium content isn't always listed on food labels. However, you can still make informed choices by opting for low-potassium versions of products when possible, like low-potassium tinned fruits and vegetables.

17. **Phosphorus Content:** Similar to potassium, phosphorus content might not always be provided on labels. In such cases, choose low-phosphorus alternatives. Fresh and unprocessed foods are generally lower in phosphorus.

18. **Protein Content:** Pay attention to the protein content, especially in packaged foods. If a product is high in protein, consider whether it aligns with your dietary restrictions.

19. **Serving Size:** Be aware of the serving size indicated on the label. It's essential for accurate nutrient calculation. If a package contains multiple servings, make sure to adjust the values accordingly.

20. **Ingredients List:** Examine the components list for additives and preservatives that may not be kidney-friendly. The fewer and simpler the components, the better.

21. **Allergen Warnings:** Check for allergen warnings if you have food allergies or sensitivities in addition to your renal diet.

22. **Fresh Produce:** When shopping for fresh produce, look for ripe, high-quality items. While potassium content may not be listed, you can generally find kidney-friendly options like apples, strawberries, and bell peppers.

23. **Meal Planning:** Before heading to the store, plan your meals and create a shopping list. This not only saves time but also helps you stay on track with your dietary goals.

By understanding how to decode food labels and being a savvy shopper, you can fill your kitchen with the right components to create delicious renal diet-friendly meals. Plus, it's a skill that will present you well beyond your culinary adventure, promoting healthier eating habits overall.

Rise and Shine with Breakfast

Breakfast is often referred to as the most important meal of the day, and it's an excellent place to start your culinary adventure. In this chapter, we'll explore a variety of renal diet-friendly breakfast recipes, each designed to provide you with a nutritious and delicious start to your day. Whether you prefer sweet or savory, we've got your mornings covered.

Sunrise Berry Oatmeal: A Hug in a Bowl

Preparation time: 5 mins

Cooking time: 10 mins

Servings: 2

Ingredients:

- 1 teacup rolled oats
- 2 teacups water
- 1 teacup mixed berries (e.g., blueberries, raspberries, and strawberries)
- 2 tbsps honey or maple syrup
- 1/4 teacup severed almonds (elective)
- 1 tsp cinnamon

Directions:

1. Inside saucepot, raise the water to a boil. Stir in the rolled oats then decrease the temp. to low. Cook for 5 mins or 'til the oats are soft.

2. Split the cooked oats into two containers.

3. Top every container with mixed berries, a spray of honey or maple syrup, severed almonds (if using), and a spray of cinnamon.

4. Present warm.

Per serving: Calories: 250kcal; Fat: 6g; Carbs: 45g; Protein: 6g; Saturated fat: 0.5g; Sugar: 15g; Fiber: 7g; Sodium: 0mg

Variation 1: Apple Cinnamon Oatmeal

Preparation time: 5 mins

Cooking time: 10 mins

Servings: 2

Ingredients:

- 1 teacup rolled oats
- 2 teacups water
- 1 apple, skinned and cubed
- 2 tbsps honey or maple syrup
- 1/4 teacup severed walnuts (elective)
- 1 tsp cinnamon

Directions:

1. Inside saucepot, raise the water to a boil. Stir in the rolled oats then decrease the temp. to low. Cook for 5 mins or 'til the oats are soft.

2. Put the cubed apple and continue cooking for 2-3 mins till the apple softens.

3. Split the cooked oats and apple solution into two containers.

4. Spray every container using honey or maple syrup, spray with severed walnuts (if using), and a dash of cinnamon.

5. Present warm.

Per serving: Calories: 270kcal; Fat: 7g; Carbs: 50g; Protein: 6g; Saturated fat: 0.5g; Sugar: 20g; Fiber: 8g; Sodium: 0mg

Variation 2: Peach and Almond Oatmeal

Preparation time: 5 mins

Cooking time: 10 mins

Servings: 2

Ingredients:

- 1 teacup rolled oats
- 2 teacups water
- 1 ripe peach, skinned and carved
- 2 tbsps honey or maple syrup
- 1/4 teacup slivered almonds (elective)
- 1 tsp vanilla extract

Directions:

1. Inside saucepot, raise the water to a boil. Stir in the rolled oats then decrease the temp. to low. Cook for 5 mins or 'til the oats are soft.

2. Put the carved peach then cook for an extra 2-3 mins till the peach is soft.

3. Split the cooked oats and peach solution into two containers.

4. Spray every container using honey or maple syrup, spray with slivered almonds (if using), and include a dash of vanilla extract.

5. Present warm.

Per serving: Calories: 260kcal; Fat: 7g; Carbs: 45g; Protein: 6g; Saturated fat: 0.5g; Sugar: 18g; Fiber: 7g; Sodium: 0mg

Banana Muffins: Morning Comfort in Every Bite

Preparation time: 10 mins

Cooking time: 20 mins

Servings: 12 muffins

Ingredients:

• 2 ripe bananas, mashed

• 1/4 teacup unsweetened applesauce

• 1/4 teacup honey (or a sugar substitute if needed)

• 1/4 teacup vegetable oil

• 2 big eggs

• 1 tsp vanilla extract

• 1 1/2 teacups all-purpose flour

• 1 tsp baking soda

• 1/2 tsp baking powder

• 1/2 tsp cinnamon

• 1/4 tsp salt

Directions:

1. Warm up oven to 350 deg. F then line your muffin tin using paper liners.

2. Inside a blending container, blend the mashed bananas, applesauce, honey (or sugar substitute), vegetable oil, eggs, and vanilla extract. Blend thoroughly.

3. Inside a distinct container, whisk collectively your baking soda, flour, baking powder, cinnamon, and salt.

4. Slowly include dry components to banana solution and stir till just blended.

5. Spoon batter into your muffin teacups, filling each around 2/3 full.

6. Bake in to your warmed up oven for approximately 20 mins or 'til a toothpick immersed into a muffin comes out clean.

7. Let muffins to cool in the tin for a couple of mins, then transfer them to a wire stand to cool entirely.

Per serving: Calories: 140kcal; Fat: 5g; Carbs: 24g; Protein: 2g; Saturated fat: 0.5g; Sugar: 10g; Fiber: 1g; Sodium: 150mg

Variation 1: Blueberry Banana Muffins

Preparation time: 10 mins

Cooking time: 25 mins

Servings: 12 muffins

Ingredients:

- 2 ripe bananas, mashed
- 1/4 teacup unsweetened applesauce
- 1/4 teacup honey (or a sugar substitute if needed)
- 1/4 teacup vegetable oil
- 2 big eggs
- 1 tsp vanilla extract
- 1 1/2 teacups all-purpose flour
- 1 tsp baking soda
- 1/2 tsp baking powder
- 1/2 tsp cinnamon
- 1/4 tsp salt
- 1 teacup fresh or frozen blueberries

Directions:

1. Warm up oven to 350 deg. F then line your muffin tin using paper liners.

2. Inside a blending container, blend the mashed bananas, applesauce, honey (or sugar substitute), vegetable oil, eggs, and vanilla extract. Blend thoroughly.

3. Inside a distinct container, whisk collectively baking powder, baking soda, flour, cinnamon, and salt.

4. Slowly include dry components to banana solution and stir till just blended.

5. Gently wrap in the blueberries.

6. Spoon batter into your muffin teacups, filling each around 2/3 full.

7. Bake in to your warmed up oven for approximately 25 mins or 'til a toothpick immersed into a muffin comes out clean.

8. Let muffins to cool in the tin for a couple of mins, then transfer them to a wire stand to cool entirely.

Per serving: Calories: 140kcal; Fat: 5g; Carbs: 24g; Protein: 2g; Saturated fat: 0.5g; Sugar: 10g; Fiber: 1g; Sodium: 150mg

Variation 2: Cinnamon Walnut Banana Muffins

Preparation time: 10 mins

Cooking time: 20 mins

Servings: 12 muffins

Ingredients:

- 2 ripe bananas, mashed
- 1/4 teacup unsweetened applesauce
- 1/4 teacup honey (or a sugar substitute if needed)
- 1/4 teacup vegetable oil
- 2 big eggs
- 1 tsp vanilla extract
- 1 1/2 teacups all-purpose flour
- 1 tsp baking soda
- 1/2 tsp baking powder
- 1/2 tsp cinnamon
- 1/4 tsp salt
- 1/2 teacup severed walnuts (elective)

Directions:

1. Warm up oven to 350 deg. F then line your muffin tin using paper liners.

2. Inside a blending container, blend the mashed bananas, applesauce, honey (or sugar substitute), vegetable oil, eggs, and vanilla extract. Blend thoroughly.

3. Inside a distinct container, whisk collectively baking powder, baking soda, flour, cinnamon, and salt.

4. Slowly include dry components to banana solution and stir till just blended.

5. If you are using walnuts, wrap them into the batter.

6. Spoon batter into your muffin teacups, filling each around 2/3 full.

7. Bake in to your warmed up oven for approximately 20 mins or 'til a toothpick immersed into a muffin comes out clean.

8. Let muffins to cool in the tin for a couple of mins, then transfer them to a wire stand to cool entirely.

Per serving: Calories: 160kcal; Fat: 7g; Carbs: 24g; Protein: 3g; Saturated fat: 0.5g; Sugar: 10g; Fiber: 1g; Sodium: 150mg

Veggie-Loaded Scrambled Eggs: A Colorful Morning Plate

Preparation time: 5 mins

Cooking time: 10 mins

Servings: 2

Ingredients:

• 4 big eggs

• 1/4 teacup cubed bell peppers

• 1/4 teacup cubed zucchini

• 1/4 teacup cubed onion

• 1/4 teacup cubed tomatoes (without seeds)

• 1/4 teacup low-sodium vegetable broth

• Salt and pepper as required

• 1 tbsp olive oil

• Fresh parsley for garnish (elective)

Directions:

1. In non-stick griddle, warm the olive oil in a middling temp.

2. Put the cubed onions, bell peppers, and zucchini. Sauté for 3-4 mins or 'til they start to soften.

3. Put the cubed tomatoes then cook for an extra 2 mins.

4. Inside a distinct container, beat the eggs, and flavour with a tweak of salt and pepper.

5. Pour the whisked eggs over the sautéed vegetables.

6. Gently scramble the eggs, mixing irregularly 'til they're cooked to your desired level of doneness.

7. If the eggs start to stick, you can include a little low-sodium vegetable broth to keep them moist.

8. Once the eggs are done, garnish with fresh parsley if anticipated.

Per serving: Calories: 180kcal; Fat: 12g; Carbs: 5g; Protein: 13g; Saturated fat: 2g; Sugar: 2g; Fiber: 1g; Sodium: 180mg

Variation 1: Spinach and Mushroom Scramble

Preparation time: 5 mins

Cooking time: 10 mins

Servings: 2

Ingredients:

• 4 big eggs

• 1 teacup fresh spinach leaves, severed

• 1 teacup carved mushrooms

- 1/4 teacup cubed onion
- 1/4 teacup low-sodium vegetable broth
- Salt and pepper as required
- 1 tbsp olive oil

Directions:

1. In non-stick griddle, warm the olive oil in a middling temp.

2. Put the cubed onions and carved mushrooms. Sauté for 4-5 mins or 'til the mushrooms release their moisture and start to brown.

3. Put the severed spinach and sauté for an extra 2 mins till it wilts.

4. Inside a distinct container, beat the eggs, and flavour with a tweak of salt and pepper.

5. Pour the whisked eggs over the sautéed vegetables.

6. Gently scramble the eggs, mixing irregularly 'til they're cooked to your desired level of doneness.

7. If the eggs start to stick, you can include a little low-sodium vegetable broth to keep them moist.

Per serving: Calories: 160kcal; Fat: 10g; Carbs: 5g; Protein: 13g; Saturated fat: 2g; Sugar: 2g; Fiber: 2g; Sodium: 200mg

Variation 2: Tomato and Basil Scramble

Preparation time: 5 mins

Cooking time: 10 mins

Servings: 2

Ingredients:

- 4 big eggs
- 1 teacup cubed fresh tomatoes (without seeds)
- 2 tbsps fresh basil leaves, severed
- 1/4 teacup cubed onion
- Salt and pepper as required
- 1 tbsp olive oil

Directions:

1. In non-stick griddle, warm the olive oil in a middling temp.

2. Put the cubed onions and sauté for 2-3 mins 'til they soften.

3. Put the cubed tomatoes and severed basil. Sauté for an extra 2 mins.

4. Inside a distinct container, beat the eggs, and flavour with a tweak of salt and pepper.

5. Pour the whisked eggs over the sautéed vegetables.

6. Gently scramble the eggs, mixing irregularly 'til they're cooked to your desired level of doneness.

Per serving: Calories: 140kcal; Fat: 8g; Carbs: 6g; Protein: 11g; Saturated fat: 2g; Sugar: 3g; Fiber: 2g; Sodium: 170mg

Oatmeal with Fresh Berries

Preparation time: 5 mins

Cooking time: 5 mins

Servings: 1

Ingredients:

- 1/2 teacup old-fashioned oats
- 1 teacup water
- 1/2 teacup fresh mixed berries (strawberries, blueberries, raspberries)

- 1 tbsp honey (elective, for sweetness)

- 1/4 tsp cinnamon (elective, for flavor)

Directions:

1. Inside saucepot, bring water to a boil.

2. Put the oats then cook for 5 mins, mixing irregularly 'til they reach your anticipated uniformity.

3. Take out from temp. and transfer the oatmeal to a container.

4. Top with fresh berries then spray with honey if anticipated. Spray with a tweak of cinnamon for added flavor.

5. Present hot.

Per serving: Calories: 250kcal; Fat: 2g; Carbs: 55g; Protein: 5g; Saturated fat: 0.5g; Sugar: 13g; Fiber: 8g; Sodium: 5mg

Quinoa Breakfast Bowl

Preparation time: 10 mins

Cooking time: 15 mins

Servings: 2

Ingredients:

- 1/2 teacup quinoa

- 1 teacup water

- 1/2 teacup carved strawberries

- 1/2 teacup carved kiwi

- 2 tbsps severed almonds

- 1 tbsp honey (elective, for sweetness)

Directions:

1. Wash the quinoa thoroughly under cold water.

2. Inside saucepot, blend the washed quinoa and water. Boil, then decrease temp. to simmer, cover, then cook for 15 mins or 'til the quinoa is cooked and the water is immersed.

3. Split the cooked quinoa among two containers.

4. Top with carved strawberries, kiwi, and severed almonds.

5. Spray with honey if anticipated.

6. Present warm.

Per serving: Calories: 280kcal; Fat: 6g; Carbs: 49g; Protein: 8g; Saturated fat: 0.5g; Sugar: 10g; Fiber: 6g; Sodium: 5mg

Buckwheat Pancakes with Blueberry Compote

Preparation time: 10 mins

Cooking time: 15 mins

Servings: 2-3

Ingredients:

For Pancakes:

- 1/2 teacup buckwheat flour

- 1/2 teacup milk (use a milk substitute if necessary)

- 1 egg

- 1 tbsp honey (elective, for sweetness)

- 1/2 tsp baking powder

- Cooking spray or a small amount of oil for cooking

For Blueberry Compote:

- 1 teacup fresh or frozen blueberries

- 1 tbsp honey (elective, for sweetness)

Directions:

For Pancakes:

1. Inside a blending container, whisk collectively the buckwheat flour, milk, egg, honey, and baking powder till you have a smooth batter.

2. Warm a non-stick griddle in a middling temp. and mildly oil using cooking spray or oil.

3. Place 1/4 teacup of your pancake batter onto the griddle for every pancake.

4. Cook 'til bubbles form on the surface, then flip then cook the other side till golden brown.

5. Repeat with the rest of the batter.

For Blueberry Compote:

6. Inside small saucepan, blend the blueberries and honey.

7. Cook in a middling temp., mixing irregularly, 'til the blueberries break down then the solution thickens (around 5-7 mins).

8. Present the pancakes with the blueberry compote on top.

Per serving: Calories: 245kcal; Fat: 4g; Carbs: 48g; Protein: 7g; Saturated fat: 1g; Sugar: 16g; Fiber: 6g; Sodium: 45mg

---

Poached Egg on Whole Grain Toast

Preparation time: 5 mins

Cooking time: 5 mins

Servings: 1

Ingredients:

• 1 big egg

• 1 slice of whole grain bread

• 1/2 tsp white vinegar (for poaching)

• Salt and pepper as required

Directions:

1. Fill a small saucepan with water and bring it to a gentle simmer.

2. Include white vinegar to the simmering water (this helps the egg white coagulate).

3. Carefully crack egg into a small container.

4. Create a gentle whirlpool in simmering water using a spoon, then carefully slide the egg into the center of the whirlpool.

5. Poach egg for 3-4 mins for a runny yolk, or longer if anticipated.

6. While the egg is poaching, toast the whole grain bread.

7. Take out poached egg with a slotted spoon, allowing extra water to drain.

8. Put the poached egg on top of the toasted bread.

9. Flavour with salt and pepper as required.

10. Present instantly.

Per serving: Calories: 170kcal; Fat: 6g; Carbs: 17g; Protein: 12g; Saturated fat: 2g; Sugar: 1g; Fiber: 2g; Sodium: 150mg

---

Low-Sodium Breakfast Burrito

Preparation time: 10 mins

Cooking time: 10 mins

Servings: 2

Ingredients:

For the Filling:

• 4 big eggs, whisked

- 1/4 teacup cubed bell peppers
- 1/4 teacup cubed onions
- 1/4 teacup low-sodium salsa
- Salt and pepper as required
- Cooking spray

For the Burrito:

- 2 whole grain tortillas
- 1/4 teacup low-fat teared up cheese (elective)

Directions:

1. In non-stick griddle, heat cooking spray in a middling temp.

2. Include cubed bell peppers and onions and sauté till softened.

3. Pour the whisked eggs over the sautéed vegetables and scramble them till cooked.

4. Flavour with salt and pepper as required.

5. Warm the whole grain tortillas in the microwave or on a dry griddle.

6. Split scrambled eggs among the two tortillas.

7. Top with low-sodium salsa and elective low-fat teared up cheese.

8. Roll the tortillas into burritos and present.

Per serving: Calories: 240kcal; Fat: 10g; Carbs: 23g; Protein: 15g; Saturated fat: 3g; Sugar: 4g; Fiber: 5g; Sodium: 200mg

---

Fresh Fruit Salad with Honey Yogurt Dressing

Preparation time: 10 mins

Cooking time: 0 mins

Servings: 2

Ingredients:

For the Salad:

- 1 teacup mixed fresh fruits (e.g., berries, melon, apple slices)

- 1/4 teacup grapes, divided
- 1/4 teacup pineapple chunks

For the Dressing:

- 1/4 teacup plain low-fat yogurt
- 1 tbsp honey
- 1/4 tsp vanilla extract

Directions:

1. Inside a container, blend the mixed fresh fruits, grapes, and pineapple chunks.

2. Inside a distinct container, whisk collectively the plain low-fat yogurt, honey, and vanilla extract to create the dressing.

3. Spray the honey yogurt dressing over the fruit salad then carefully shake to cover.

4. Present instantly.

Per serving: Calories: 150kcal; Fat: 1g; Carbs: 37g; Protein: 2g; Saturated fat: 0g; Sugar: 31g; Fiber: 3g; Sodium: 35mg

Midday Meals to Fuel Your Day

Lunch is a pivotal meal in your daily culinary journey, providing the energy and nourishment you need to carry on with your day. In this chapter, we'll explore a selection of renal diet-friendly midday meals that are not only delicious but also filling. These recipes will keep you and your trusted friend satisfied and energized throughout the day.

Sunny Tuna Salad Sandwich: A Picnic Favorite

Preparation time: 15 mins

Cooking time: 0 mins

Servings: 2

Ingredients:

- 1 tin of low-sodium tuna, drained
- 1/2 teacup cubed cucumber
- 1/4 teacup cubed red bell pepper
- 2 tbsps severed fresh parsley
- 2 tbsps light mayonnaise
- 1 tbsp Dijon mustard
- 1/2 tsp lemon juice
- Salt and pepper as required
- 4 slices of whole-grain bread
- Lettuce leaves and carved cucumber (for garnish, elective)

Directions:

1. Inside a blending container, blend the drained tuna, cubed cucumber, cubed red bell pepper, and severed parsley.

2. Inside a distinct small container, mix the mayonnaise, Dijon mustard, and lemon juice. Include this solution to the tuna and vegetables, and stir well to blend.

3. Flavour with salt and pepper as required.

4. Place lettuce leaves and carved cucumber on two slices of whole-grain bread.

5. Spoon the tuna salad solution onto the bread slices with lettuce and cucumber.

6. Top using ith remaining bread slices to create sandwiches.

7. Cut the sandwiches in half, and they're ready to present.

Per serving: Calories: 265kcal; Fat: 9g; Carbs: 23g; Protein: 21g; Saturated fat: 1g; Sugar: 4g; Fiber: 5g; Sodium: 367mg

Variation 1: Creamy Avocado Tuna Salad Sandwich

Preparation time: 15 mins

Cooking time: 0 mins

Servings: 2

Ingredients:

- 1 tin of low-sodium tuna, drained
- 1 ripe avocado, mashed
- 2 tbsps Greek yogurt
- 2 tsps lemon juice
- 2 tbsps severed fresh cilantro
- Salt and pepper as required
- 4 slices of whole-grain bread
- Lettuce leaves and carved tomato (for garnish, elective)

Directions:

1. Inside a blending container, blend the drained tuna, mashed avocado, Greek yogurt, lemon juice, and severed cilantro.

2. Stir well 'til all components are thoroughly mixed.

3. Flavour with salt and pepper as required.

4. Place lettuce leaves and carved tomato on two slices of whole-grain bread.

5. Spoon the creamy avocado tuna salad solution onto the bread slices with lettuce and tomato.

6. Top using the rest of the bread slices to create sandwiches.

7. Cut the sandwiches in half, and they're ready to present.

Per serving: Calories: 307kcal; Fat: 16g; Carbs: 26g; Protein: 17g; Saturated fat: 2g; Sugar: 4g; Fiber: 8g; Sodium: 327mg

Variation 2: Zesty Lemon Tuna Salad Wrap

Preparation time: 15 mins

Cooking time: 0 mins

Servings: 2

Ingredients:

- 1 tin of low-sodium tuna, drained
- 1/4 teacup cubed red onion
- 1/4 teacup cubed celery
- 1/4 teacup cubed green bell pepper
- 1/4 teacup severed fresh parsley
- 2 tbsps light mayonnaise
- 2 tsps lemon zest
- 2 tbsps lemon juice
- Salt and pepper as required
- 2 big whole-grain tortillas
- Lettuce leaves and finely carved red cabbage (for garnish, elective)

Directions:

1. Inside a blending container, blend the drained tuna, cubed red onion, cubed celery, cubed green bell pepper, and severed parsley.

2. Inside a distinct small container, mix the mayonnaise, lemon zest, and lemon juice. Include this solution to the tuna and vegetables, and stir well to blend.

3. Flavour with salt and pepper as required.

4. Warm the whole-grain tortillas briefly, if anticipated.

5. Lay out the tortillas, and place lettuce leaves and finely carved red cabbage on each.

6. Spoon the zesty lemon tuna salad solution onto the tortillas with lettuce and cabbage.

7. Roll up the tortillas, folding in the sides to create wraps.

8. Slice the wraps in half, and they're ready to present.

Per serving: Calories: 295kcal; Fat: 12g; Carbs: 34g; Protein: 18g; Saturated fat: 2g; Sugar: 5g; Fiber: 7g; Sodium: 329mg

Heartwarming Vegetable Soup: A Hug in a Bowl

Preparation time: 15 mins

Cooking time: 30 mins

Servings: 4

Ingredients:

- 1 tbsp olive oil
- 1 medium onion, severed
- 2 carrots, skinned and cubed
- 2 celery stalks, cubed
- 2 pieces garlic, crushed
- 4 teacups low-sodium vegetable broth
- 1 teacup green beans, that is cut into bite-sized pieces
- 1 teacup zucchini, cubed
- 1 teacup butternut squash, cubed
- 1 tsp dried thyme
- 1 tsp dried oregano

33

- Salt and pepper as required
- Fresh parsley for garnish (elective)

Directions:

1. Inside big pot, warm the olive oil in a middling temp. Put the severed onion, carrots, and celery. Sauté for 5 mins or 'til the vegetables start to soften.

2. Put the crushed garlic and sauté for an extra min.

3. Pour in vegetable broth and include the green beans, zucchini, and butternut squash.

4. Stir in the dried thyme and oregano. Flavour with salt and pepper as required.

5. Boil the soup, then decrease the temp. to a simmer. Cover then cook for 20-25 mins or 'til the vegetables are soft.

6. Scoop the hot vegetable soup into containers, garnish with fresh parsley if anticipated, and present.

Per serving: Calories: 120kcal; Fat: 3g; Carbs: 22g; Protein: 3g; Saturated fat: 0.5g; Sugar: 6g; Fiber: 5g; Sodium: 450mg

Variation 1: Creamy Potato Vegetable Soup

Preparation time: 15 mins

Cooking time: 30 mins

Servings: 4

Ingredients:

- 2 medium potatoes, skinned and cubed
- 1 carrot, skinned and cubed
- 1 celery stalk, cubed
- 1 small onion, severed
- 4 teacups low-sodium vegetable broth
- 1 teacup green peas

- 1/2 teacup cauliflower florets
- 1/2 teacup low-fat sour cream
- 1 tsp dried thyme
- Salt and pepper as required
- Fresh chives for garnish (elective)

Directions:

1. Inside big pot, blend the potatoes, carrot, celery, and onion with the vegetable broth. Boil then decrease the temp. to simmer. Cook for 20-25 mins or 'til the vegetables are soft.

2. Use blender to puree soup 'til smooth.

3. Return pureed soup to the pot then include the green peas, cauliflower, dried thyme, salt, and pepper. Cook for an extra 5-7 mins till the peas and cauliflower are soft.

4. Stir in the low-fat sour cream, and heat the soup for an extra 2-3 mins.

5. Scoop the hot creamy potato vegetable soup into containers, garnish with fresh chives if anticipated, and present.

Per serving: Calories: 160kcal; Fat: 4g; Carbs: 26g; Protein: 5g; Saturated fat: 2g; Sugar: 6g; Fiber: 6g; Sodium: 350mg

Variation 2: Creamy Asparagus Soup

Preparation time: 10 mins

Cooking time: 20 mins

Servings: 4

Ingredients:

- 1 bunch asparagus, clipped and severed
- 1 small onion, severed
- 2 pieces garlic, crushed
- 4 teacups low-sodium vegetable broth
- 1 teacup cauliflower florets

- 1/2 teacup low-fat plain Greek yogurt
- 1 tsp dried tarragon
- Salt and pepper as required
- Lemon zest for garnish (elective)

Directions:

1. Inside big pot, sauté the severed onion and asparagus in a middling temp. 'til they start to soften, around 5 mins. Put the crushed garlic and sauté for an extra min.

2. Pour in vegetable broth and include the cauliflower florets. Boil, then decrease the temp. to simmer. Cover then cook for 15 mins or 'til the vegetables are soft.

3. Use blender to puree the soup 'til smooth.

4. Return pureed soup to the pot then stir in the low-fat plain Greek yogurt, dried tarragon, salt, and pepper. Heat for an extra 2-3 mins.

5. Scoop the hot creamy asparagus soup into containers, garnish with lemon zest if anticipated, then present.

Per serving: Calories: 90kcal; Fat: 2g; Carbs: 14g; Protein: 6g; Saturated fat: 1g; Sugar: 6g; Fiber: 4g; Sodium: 450mg

---

Crisp and Fresh Chicken Caesar: A Lunchtime Classic

Preparation time: 15 mins

Cooking time: 15 mins

Servings: 2

Ingredients:

- 2 boneless, skinless chicken breasts
- 2 teacups Romaine lettuce, severed

- 1/4 teacup cherry tomatoes, divided
- 2 tbsps low-sodium Caesar dressing
- 1/4 teacup croutons
- 1 tbsp grated Parmesan cheese (elective)

Directions:

1. Flavour chicken breasts with a tweak of black pepper and grill or pan-fry them till fully cooked, about 6-7 mins on all sides. Ensure chicken reaches an internal temp. of 165 deg.F. Slice the cooked chicken into thin strips.

2. Inside big container, blend the severed Romaine lettuce, cherry tomatoes, then cooked chicken strips.

3. Spray the low-sodium Caesar dressing over the salad and shake till well covered.

4. Spray the croutons on top and, if anticipated, include a tbsp of your grated Parmesan cheese for extra flavor.

5. Present instantly and relish!

Per serving: Calories: 300kcal; Fat: 9g; Carbs: 14g; Protein: 40g; Saturated fat: 2g; Sugar: 2g; Fiber: 2g; Sodium: 450mg

Variation 1: Grilled Shrimp Caesar Salad

Preparation time: 15 mins

Cooking time: 10 mins

Servings: 2

Ingredients:

- 12 big shrimp, skinned and deveined
- 2 teacups Romaine lettuce, severed
- 1/4 teacup cherry tomatoes, divided
- 2 tbsps low-sodium Caesar dressing
- 1/4 teacup croutons

• 1 tbsp grated Parmesan cheese (elective)

Directions:

1. Flavour the shrimp with a tweak of black pepper and grill or pan-fry them 'til they turn pink and opaque, approximately 2-3 mins on all sides.

2. Inside big container, blend the severed Romaine lettuce, cherry tomatoes, and grilled shrimp.

3. Spray the low-sodium Caesar dressing over the salad and shake till well covered.

4. Spray the croutons on top and, if anticipated, include a tbsp of your grated Parmesan cheese for extra flavor.

5. Present instantly for a delicious and low-phosphorus shrimp Caesar salad.

Per serving: Calories: 250kcal; Fat: 7g; Carbs: 12g; Protein: 30g; Saturated fat: 2g; Sugar: 2g; Fiber: 2g; Sodium: 450mg

Variation 2: Avocado and Turkey Caesar Salad

Preparation time: 15 mins

Cooking time: 0 mins

Servings: 2

Ingredients:

• 8 oz. cooked turkey breast, carved

• 2 teacups Romaine lettuce, severed

• 1/4 teacup cherry tomatoes, divided

• 2 tbsps low-sodium Caesar dressing

• 1/4 teacup croutons

• 1/2 ripe avocado, carved

Directions:

1. Inside big container, blend the severed Romaine lettuce, cherry tomatoes, and carved turkey breast.

2. Spray the low-sodium Caesar dressing over the salad and shake till well covered.

3. Put the avocado slices then carefully mix them into the salad.

4. Spray the croutons on top, providing a delicious crunch.

5. Present instantly for a unique and low-phosphorus avocado and turkey Caesar salad.

Per serving: Calories: 320kcal; Fat: 11g; Carbs: 17g; Protein: 35g; Saturated fat: 2g; Sugar: 3g; Fiber: 6g; Sodium: 450mg

Grilled Chicken and Vegetable Salad

Preparation time: 15 mins

Cooking time: 15 mins

Servings: 2

Ingredients:

For the Salad:

• 2 boneless, skinless chicken breasts

• 4 teacups mixed salad greens (lettuce, spinach, arugula, etc.)

• 1 teacup cherry tomatoes, divided

• 1/2 cucumber, carved

• 1/4 red onion, finely carved

• 1/4 teacup low-fat feta cheese (elective)

For the Dressing:

• 2 tbsps olive oil

• 1 tbsp balsamic vinegar

• 1 tsp Dijon mustard

- Salt and pepper as required

Directions:

1. Warm up your grill or your stovetop grill pan to med-high temp.

2. Flavour chicken breasts with salt and pepper.

3. Grill the chicken for 6-7 mins on all sides or 'til fully cooked.

4. Let the chicken rest for a couple of mins, then slice it into thin strips.

5. Inside big salad container, blend the salad greens, cherry tomatoes, cucumber, and red onion.

6. Top the salad with grilled chicken and feta cheese if anticipated.

7. Inside a distinct container, whisk collectively the salt, olive oil, balsamic vinegar, Dijon mustard, and pepper to create the dressing.

8. Transfer dressing over the salad, shake to blend, and present.

Per serving: Calories: 350kcal; Fat: 17g; Carbs: 11g; Protein: 37g; Saturated fat: 4g; Sugar: 6g; Fiber: 3g; Sodium: 280mg

Turkey and Avocado Wrap

Preparation time: 10 mins

Cooking time: 0 mins

Servings: 2

Ingredients:

- 4 big whole grain tortillas
- 8 slices low-sodium turkey breast
- 1 avocado, carved
- 1 teacup mixed salad greens
- 1/4 teacup low-fat ranch dressing
- Salt and pepper as required

Directions:

1. Lay out the whole grain tortillas.

2. Disperse 2 slices of low-sodium turkey breast on each tortilla.

3. Include avocado slices and mixed salad greens on top of the turkey.

4. Spray low-fat ranch dressing evenly over each wrap.

5. Flavour with salt and pepper as required.

6. Roll up the tortillas into wraps and present.

Per serving: Calories: 350kcal; Fat: 16g; Carbs: 40g; Protein: 20g; Saturated fat: 3g; Sugar: 4g; Fiber: 9g; Sodium: 400mg

Quinoa and Black Bean Bowl

Preparation time: 15 mins

Cooking time: 20 mins

Servings: 2

Ingredients:

For the Bowl:

- 1 teacup cooked quinoa
- 1 teacup tinned low-sodium black beans, that is drained and washed
- 1/2 teacup corn kernels
- 1/2 red bell pepper, cubed
- 1/4 teacup severed fresh cilantro

For the Dressing:

- 2 tbsps olive oil

- 2 tbsps lime juice

- 1 piece garlic, crushed

- Salt and pepper as required

Directions:

1. Inside big container, blend the cooked quinoa, black beans, corn, red bell pepper, and cilantro.

2. Inside a distinct container, whisk collectively the salt, crushed garlic, olive oil, lime juice, and pepper to create the dressing.

3. Transfer dressing over the quinoa and black bean solution and shake to blend.

4. Present warm or cold.

Per serving: Calories: 320kcal; Fat: 11g; Carbs: 50g; Protein: 10g; Saturated fat: 1.5g; Sugar: 4g; Fiber: 9g; Sodium: 150mg

---

Baked White Fish with Lemon and Herbs

Preparation time: 10 mins

Cooking time: 20 mins

Servings: 2

Ingredients:

For the Fish:

- 2 white fish fillets (e.g., cod or tilapia)

- 2 tbsps fresh lemon juice

- 1 tsp olive oil

- 1/2 tsp dried oregano

- Salt and pepper as required

For Garnish:

- Fresh parsley, severed

- Lemon wedges

Directions:

1. Warm up oven to 375 deg.F.

2. Place fish fillets in a baking dish.

3. Inside small container, whisk collectively the salt, lemon juice, olive oil, dried oregano, and pepper.

4. Spray the lemon herb solution over the fish fillets.

5. Cover the baking dish using foil and bake for 15-20 mins or 'til the fish is fully cooked then flakes simply with a fork.

6. Garnish using fresh severed parsley and present with lemon wedges.

Per serving: Calories: 150kcal; Fat: 3g; Carbs: 1g; Protein: 30g; Saturated fat: 0.5g; Sugar: 0g; Fiber: 0g; Sodium: 90mg

---

Tofu Stir-Fry with Mixed Vegetables

Preparation time: 15 mins

Cooking time: 15 mins

Servings: 2

Ingredients:

For the Stir-Fry:

- 8 oz firm tofu, cubed

- 1 teacup mixed vegetables (bell peppers, broccoli, snap peas, carrots)

- 1 tbsp low-sodium soy sauce

- 1 tbsp low-sodium stir-fry sauce

- 1 tbsp vegetable oil

For Garnish:

- Sesame seeds (elective)

- Chopped green onions (elective)

Directions:

1. In non-stick griddle or wok, heat the vegetable oil in a med-high temp.

2. Put the tofu cubes and stir-fry 'til they are golden brown.

3. Take out the tofu and put it away.

4. In the same pan, include the mixed vegetables and stir-fry 'til they are crisp-soft.

5. Return the tofu to the pan and include the low-sodium soy sauce and stir-fry sauce. Shake to blend and heat through.

6. Garnish using sesame seeds and severed green onions if anticipated.

7. Present hot over cooked brown rice or whole grain noodles.

Per serving: Calories: 250kcal; Fat: 14g; Carbs: 12g; Protein: 18g; Saturated fat: 2g; Sugar: 3g; Fiber: 3g; Sodium: 300mg

Couscous Salad with Fresh Herbs

Preparation time: 15 mins

Cooking time: 5 mins

Servings: 4

Ingredients:

For the Salad:

• 1 teacup whole wheat couscous

• 1 1/4 teacups water

• 1 teacup cubed cucumbers

• 1 teacup cubed tomatoes

• 1/4 teacup severed fresh parsley

• 1/4 teacup severed fresh mint

• 1/4 teacup severed green onions

For the Dressing:

• 3 tbsps olive oil

• 2 tbsps fresh lemon juice

• 1 piece garlic, crushed

• Salt and pepper as required

Directions:

1. Inside saucepot, raise the water to a boil.

2. Stir in the couscous, cover, and take out from temp.. Let it rest for 5 mins, then fluff using a fork.

3. Inside big container, blend the cooked couscous, cubed cucumbers, tomatoes, fresh parsley, fresh mint, and green onions.

4. Inside a distinct container, whisk collectively the salt, lemon juice, crushed garlic, olive oil, and pepper to create the dressing.

5. Transfer dressing over the couscous salad and shake to blend.

6. Present at room temp. or chilled.

Per serving: Calories: 220kcal; Fat: 8g; Carbs: 33g; Protein: 5g; Saturated fat: 1g; Sugar: 2g; Fiber: 5g; Sodium: 15mg

Dinners to Come Home To

Dinner is a time to unwind, relax, and savor a comforting meal after a long day. In this chapter, we'll explore a range of renal diet-friendly dinner recipes that are not only delicious but also satisfying. These recipes will turn your evening meals into a delightful experience you and your trusted friend can look forward to.

Homestyle Beef Stew: Comfort in Every Bite

Preparation time: 15 mins

Cooking time: 2 hrs

Servings: 4

Ingredients:

- 1 lb. lean beef stew meat, that is cut into cubes
- 1 onion, cubed
- 2 carrots, skinned and severed
- 2 celery stalks, severed
- 2 teacups low-sodium beef broth
- 1 teacup water
- 1 teacup potatoes, skinned and cubed
- 1 teacup green beans, clipped then cut into bite-sized pieces
- 1 bay leaf
- 1/2 tsp dried thyme
- Salt and black pepper as required
- 1 tbsp olive oil

Directions:

1. Inside big pot, warm the olive oil in a middling temp. Put the cubed onion and beef cubes. Sauté till the beef is browned on all sides.

2. Put the carrots, celery, and potatoes to the pot. Sauté for a couple of mins till the vegetables begin to soften.

3. Pour in the low-sodium beef broth and water. Stir in the bay leaf, thyme, salt, and black pepper. Bring the solution to a boil.

4. Decrease temp., cover then simmer for 1.5 to 2 hrs, or 'til the beef is soft and the flavors meld together.

5. About 20 mins prior to presenting, place green beans to the pot and continue to simmer 'til they are soft yet crisp.

6. Take out bay leaf and adjust the seasoning if needed.

7. Present your delicious and kidney-friendly homestyle beef stew hot and relish!

Per serving: Calories: 250kcal; Fat: 7g; Carbs: 20g; Protein: 25g; Saturated fat: 2g; Sugar: 5g; Fiber: 4g; Sodium: 300mg

Variation 1: Chicken and Vegetable Stew

Preparation time: 15 mins

Cooking time: 1.5 hrs

Servings: 4

Ingredients:

- 1 lb. boneless, that is skinless chicken thighs, cut into bite-sized pieces
- 1 onion, cubed
- 2 carrots, skinned and severed
- 2 celery stalks, severed
- 2 teacups low-sodium chicken broth
- 1 teacup water
- 1 teacup potatoes, skinned and cubed
- 1 teacup green beans, clipped then cut into bite-sized pieces
- 1 bay leaf
- 1/2 tsp dried thyme
- Salt and black pepper as required
- 1 tbsp olive oil

Directions:

1. Follow the same cooking steps as the beef stew, replacing the beef with chicken. Sauté the

chicken till it's fully cooked and no longer pink inside.

2. Continue with the same vegetable and seasoning steps, simmering till the chicken is soft and the stew is flavorful.

3. Put the green beans in the last 20 mins of cooking.

4. Present your kidney-friendly chicken and vegetable stew hot and relish!

Per serving: Calories: 230kcal; Fat: 8g; Carbs: 20g; Protein: 20g; Saturated fat: 2g; Sugar: 5g; Fiber: 4g; Sodium: 290mg

Variation 2: Turkey and Mushroom Stew

Preparation time: 15 mins

Cooking time: 2 hrs

Servings: 4

Ingredients:

- 1 lb. ground turkey
- 1 onion, cubed
- 2 carrots, skinned and severed
- 2 celery stalks, severed
- 2 teacups low-sodium vegetable broth
- 1 teacup water
- 1 teacup mushrooms, carved
- 1 teacup potatoes, skinned and cubed
- 1 bay leaf
- 1/2 tsp dried thyme
- Salt and black pepper as required
- 1 tbsp olive oil

Directions:

1. Inside big pot, warm the olive oil in a middling temp. Put the cubed onion and ground turkey. Cook 'til the turkey is browned.

2. Put the carrots, celery, and mushrooms. Sauté for a couple of mins till the vegetables begin to soften.

3. Pour in the low-sodium vegetable broth and water. Stir in the bay leaf, thyme, salt, and black pepper. Bring the solution to a boil.

4. Decrease temp., cover then simmer for 1.5 to 2 hrs, or 'til the flavors meld together and the stew thickens.

5. About 20 mins prior to presenting, include the potatoes and continue to simmer 'til they are soft.

6. Take out bay leaf then adjust the seasoning if needed.

7. Present your kidney-friendly turkey and mushroom stew hot and relish!

Per serving: Calories: 230kcal; Fat: 7g; Carbs: 20g; Protein: 22g; Saturated fat: 2g; Sugar: 5g; Fiber: 4g; Sodium: 310mg

---

Salmon with Zesty Lemon Herb Drizzle: A Dinner Date Star

Preparation time: 10 mins

Cooking time: 15 mins

Servings: 2

Ingredients:

- 2 salmon fillets
- 1 lemon, zested and juiced
- 2 tbsps fresh parsley, finely severed
- 1 piece garlic, crushed

- 1 tbsp olive oil
- Salt and black pepper as required

Directions:

1. Warm up oven to 375 deg.F.

2. Place salmon fillets on baking sheet covered using parchment paper. Spray them using olive oil, then flavour with salt and black pepper.

3. Bake salmon in the warmed up oven for 12-15 mins, or 'til the salmon flakes simply with a fork.

4. While the salmon is baking, prepare the zesty lemon herb spray. Inside small container, blend the lemon zest, lemon juice, crushed garlic, and severed parsley.

5. When the salmon is cooked, spray the lemon herb solution over the fillets.

6. Present salmon hot with your choice of kidney-friendly side dishes.

Per serving: Calories: 300kcal; Fat: 15g; Carbs: 4g; Protein: 38g; Saturated fat: 2g; Sugar: 1g; Fiber: 2g; Sodium: 150mg

Variation 1: Baked Tilapia with Lemon Herb Drizzle

Preparation time: 10 mins

Cooking time: 12 mins

Servings: 2

Ingredients:

- 2 tilapia fillets
- 1 lemon, zested and juiced
- 2 tbsps fresh parsley, finely severed
- 1 piece garlic, crushed
- 1 tbsp olive oil
- Salt and black pepper as required

Directions:

1. Follow the same preparation and baking steps as the original salmon recipe, replacing the salmon with tilapia fillets.

2. Prepare the zesty lemon herb spray as described in the main recipe.

3. When the tilapia is cooked, spray the lemon herb solution over the fillets.

4. Present the tilapia hot with kidney-friendly sides.

Per serving: Calories: 250kcal; Fat: 12g; Carbs: 4g; Protein: 30g; Saturated fat: 2g; Sugar: 1g; Fiber: 2g; Sodium: 160mg

Variation 2: Lemon Herb Grilled Chicken

Preparation time: 10 mins

Cooking time: 15 mins

Servings: 2

Ingredients:

- 2 boneless, skinless chicken breasts
- 1 lemon, zested and juiced
- 2 tbsps fresh parsley, finely severed
- 1 piece garlic, crushed
- 1 tbsp olive oil
- Salt and black pepper as required

Directions:

1. Warm up your grill to med-high temp.

2. Flavour chicken breasts using salt and black pepper.

3. Grill the chicken for 6-8 mins on all sides or 'til fully cooked and no longer pink in the center.

4. While the chicken is grilling, prepare the zesty lemon herb spray. Inside small container, blend the lemon zest, lemon juice, crushed garlic, and severed parsley.

5. Once the chicken is cooked, spray the lemon herb solution over the breasts.

6. Present the grilled chicken hot with kidney-friendly side dishes.

Per serving: Calories: 260kcal; Fat: 10g; Carbs: 5g; Protein: 35g; Saturated fat: 2g; Sugar: 1g; Fiber: 2g; Sodium: 160mg

Vibrant Veggie Stir-Fry: A Rainbow on Your Plate

Preparation time: 15 mins

Cooking time: 10 mins

Servings: 2

Ingredients:

• 2 teacups mixed colorful bell peppers, finely carved

• 1 teacup broccoli florets

• 1 carrot, julienned

• 1 teacup snap peas, clipped

• 1 piece garlic, crushed

• 1 tbsp low-sodium soy sauce

• 1 tsp sesame oil

• 1 tbsp vegetable oil (for stir-frying)

• Sesame seeds for garnish (elective)

Directions:

1. Heat vegetable oil in big pan in a med-high temp.

2. Put the crushed garlic and stir-fry for 30 seconds till it becomes fragrant.

3. Shake in the julienned carrot, broccoli florets, and snap peas. Stir-fry for 3-4 mins 'til they start to become soft but remain crisp.

4. Put the finely carved bell peppers and continue stir-frying for an extra 2-3 mins till the veggies are soft-crisp.

5. Inside small container, blend collectively the low-sodium soy sauce and sesame oil.

6. Pour the soy sauce solution over the stir-fried vegetables and shake to blend. Cook for an extra min to heat the sauce through.

7. Present your vibrant veggie stir-fry as is or over a kidney-friendly grain like brown rice or quinoa. Garnish using sesame seeds if anticipated.

Per serving: Calories: 120kcal; Fat: 7g; Carbs: 12g; Protein: 4g; Saturated fat: 1g; Sugar: 5g; Fiber: 4g; Sodium: 200mg

Variation 1: Tofu and Snow Pea Stir-Fry

Preparation time: 15 mins

Cooking time: 10 mins

Servings: 2

Ingredients:

• 1 teacup extra-firm tofu, cubed

• 1 teacup snow peas, clipped

• 1 carrot, julienned

• 1 teacup carved mushrooms

• 1 piece garlic, crushed

• 1 tbsp low-sodium soy sauce

• 1 tsp sesame oil

• 1 tbsp vegetable oil (for stir-frying)

- Sesame seeds for garnish (elective)

Directions:

1. Press the tofu to take out extra water, cut it into cubes, and marinate it in a solution of low-sodium soy sauce and sesame oil for 15 mins.

2. Heat vegetable oil in big pan in a med-high temp.

3. Put the crushed garlic and stir-fry for 30 seconds till it becomes fragrant.

4. Shake in the julienned carrot and snow peas. Stir-fry for 3-4 mins 'til they start to become soft but remain crisp.

5. Put the carved mushrooms and marinated tofu cubes. Continue stir-frying for an extra 2-3 mins till the tofu is fully heated and the veggies are soft-crisp.

6. Present your tofu and snow pea stir-fry over kidney-friendly grains or noodles. Garnish using sesame seeds if anticipated.

Per serving: Calories: 150kcal; Fat: 9g; Carbs: 12g; Protein: 9g; Saturated fat: 1g; Sugar: 4g; Fiber: 4g; Sodium: 250mg

Variation 2: Shrimp and Asparagus Stir-Fry

Preparation time: 15 mins

Cooking time: 10 mins

Servings: 2

Ingredients:

- 8 oz. big shrimp, skinned and deveined
- 1 teacup asparagus spears, cut into bite-sized pieces
- 1 teacup bell peppers, finely carved
- 1 teacup carved zucchini
- 1 piece garlic, crushed
- 1 tbsp low-sodium soy sauce
- 1 tsp sesame oil
- 1 tbsp vegetable oil (for stir-frying)
- Sesame seeds for garnish (elective)

Directions:

1. Heat vegetable oil in big pan in a med-high temp.

2. Put the crushed garlic and stir-fry for 30 seconds till it becomes fragrant.

3. Shake in the asparagus, bell peppers, and zucchini. Stir-fry for 3-4 mins 'til they start to become soft but remain crisp.

4. Put the shrimp and continue stir-frying for an extra 2-3 mins till the shrimp turn pink and opaque.

5. Inside small container, blend collectively the low-sodium soy sauce and sesame oil.

6. Pour the soy sauce solution over the stir-fried shrimp and vegetables and shake to blend. Cook for an extra min to heat the sauce through.

7. Present your shrimp and asparagus stir-fry as is or over a kidney-friendly grain like brown rice or quinoa. Garnish using sesame seeds if anticipated.

Per serving: Calories: 160kcal; Fat: 8g; Carbs: 10g; Protein: 15g; Saturated fat: 1g; Sugar: 4g; Fiber: 4g; Sodium: 220mg

Baked Salmon with Herbed Quinoa

Preparation time: 15 mins

Cooking time: 25 mins

Servings: 2

Ingredients:

For the Salmon:

- 2 salmon fillets
- 1 tbsp olive oil
- 1 tsp dried dill
- 1/2 tsp garlic powder
- Salt and pepper as required

For the Quinoa:

- 1/2 teacup quinoa
- 1 teacup water or low-sodium chicken/vegetable broth
- 1 tbsp fresh severed parsley
- 1 tbsp fresh severed dill
- 1 lemon, zested and juiced

Directions:

For the Salmon:

1. Warm up oven to 375 deg.F.

2. Place salmon fillets on baking sheet covered using parchment paper.

3. Spray olive oil over salmon then spray with dried dill, garlic powder, salt, and pepper.

4. Bake in to your warmed up oven for 15-20 mins or 'til the salmon flakes simply with a fork.

For the Quinoa:

5. Wash the quinoa thoroughly under cold water.

6. Inside saucepot, blend the quinoa and water or broth. Boil.

7. Decrease temp., cover then simmer for 15 mins or 'til the liquid is immersed.

8. Fluff quinoa using a fork and stir in fresh severed parsley, dill, lemon zest, and lemon juice.

9. Present the baked salmon over the herbed quinoa.

Per serving: Calories: 400kcal; Fat: 17g; Carbs: 28g; Protein: 30g; Saturated fat: 2.5g; Sugar: 1g; Fiber: 3g; Sodium: 75mg

Brown Rice Pilaf with Sautéed Vegetables

Preparation time: 10 mins

Cooking time: 30 mins

Servings: 4

Ingredients:

- 1 teacup brown rice
- 2 teacups low-sodium chicken or vegetable broth
- 1 tbsp olive oil
- 1/2 onion, severed
- 1 carrot, cubed
- 1 red bell pepper, cubed
- 1/2 teacup frozen peas
- 1/4 teacup severed fresh parsley
- Salt and pepper as required

Directions:

1. Inside big saucepan, warm the olive oil in a middling temp.

2. Put the severed onion and sauté till it becomes translucent.

3. Stir in the brown rice then cook for 2-3 mins.

4. Pour in the low-sodium chicken or vegetable broth and raise to a boil.

5. Decrease temp., cover then simmer for 25-30 mins or 'til the rice is soft and the liquid is immersed.

6. While rice is cooking, heat a separate griddle in a middling temp. Put the cubed carrot and red bell pepper. Sauté 'til they become soft.

7. Stir in the frozen peas then cook 'til they are fully heated.

8. Once the rice is done, fluff it with a fork and stir in the sautéed vegetables and severed fresh parsley.

9. Flavour with salt and pepper as required.

Per serving: Calories: 250kcal; Fat: 4g; Carbs: 49g; Protein: 5g; Saturated fat: 0.5g; Sugar: 3g; Fiber: 5g; Sodium: 50mg

Turkey Meatballs with Marinara Sauce

Preparation time: 15 mins

Cooking time: 30 mins

Servings: 4

Ingredients:

- 1 lb. lean ground turkey
- 1/4 teacup whole wheat breadcrumbs
- 1/4 teacup grated Parmesan cheese
- 1/4 teacup severed fresh parsley
- 1/4 teacup finely severed onion
- 1 egg
- 1 piece garlic, crushed
- Salt and pepper as required

- For the Marinara Sauce:
- 1 tin (14 oz) low-sodium cubed tomatoes
- 1/2 tsp dried oregano
- 1/2 tsp dried basil
- 1/4 tsp garlic powder
- Salt and pepper as required

Directions:

For the Turkey Meatballs:

1. Warm up oven to 375 deg.F.

2. Inside a blending container, blend the ground turkey, breadcrumbs, grated Parmesan cheese, severed fresh parsley, severed onion, egg, crushed garlic, salt, and pepper.

3. Form solution into meatballs then put them on a baking sheet covered using parchment paper.

4. Bake in to your warmed up oven for 20-25 mins or 'til the meatballs are fully cooked and mildly browned.

For the Marinara Sauce:

5. Inside saucepot, blend the low-sodium cubed tomatoes, salt, dried oregano, dried basil, garlic powder, and pepper.

6. Simmer for 10 mins, mixing irregularly.

7. Present the turkey meatballs with marinara sauce.

Per serving: Calories: 250kcal; Fat: 10g; Carbs: 13g; Protein: 26g; Saturated fat: 3g; Sugar: 5g; Fiber: 4g; Sodium: 320mg

Grilled Vegetable Platter with Lemon Dill Sauce

Preparation time: 15 mins

Cooking time: 15 mins

Servings: 2

Ingredients:

For the Grilled Vegetables:

- 2 zucchinis, carved lengthwise
- 2 bell peppers, quartered and seeds taken out
- 1 red onion, carved into thick rounds
- 1 tbsp olive oil
- Salt and pepper as required

For the Lemon Dill Sauce:

- 1/2 teacup plain low-fat yogurt
- 1 tbsp fresh lemon juice
- 1 tsp fresh dill, severed
- 1 piece garlic, crushed
- Salt and pepper as required

Directions:

For the Grilled Vegetables:

1. Warm up your grill to med-high temp.

2. Inside a container, shake the carved zucchinis, bell peppers, and red onion with olive oil, salt, and pepper.

3. Grill vegetables for 5-7 mins on all sides or 'til they are soft and have grill marks.

For the Lemon Dill Sauce:

4. Inside small container, whisk collectively the plain low-fat yogurt, fresh lemon juice, severed dill, crushed garlic, salt, and pepper.

5. Present the grilled vegetables with the lemon dill sauce.

Per serving: Calories: 180kcal; Fat: 6g; Carbs: 24g; Protein: 8g; Saturated fat: 1g; Sugar: 10g; Fiber: 5g; Sodium: 50mg

---

| **Baked Cod with Steamed Asparagus** |

Preparation time: 10 mins

Cooking time: 20 mins

Servings: 2

Ingredients:

For the Cod:

- 2 cod fillets
- 1 tbsp olive oil
- 1 tsp dried thyme
- 1/2 tsp lemon zest
- Salt and pepper as required

For the Asparagus:

- 1 bunch asparagus, clipped
- 1 tbsp olive oil
- Salt and pepper as required

Directions:

For the Cod:

1. Warm up oven to 375 deg.F.

2. Place cod fillets on baking sheet covered using parchment paper.

3. Spray olive oil over the cod, spray with dried thyme, lemon zest, salt, and pepper.

4. Bake in to your warmed up oven for 15-20 mins or 'til the cod flakes simply with a fork.

For the Asparagus:

5. Steam the clipped asparagus for 3-5 mins 'til they are soft-crisp.

6. Spray olive oil over the steamed asparagus and flavour with salt and pepper.

7. Present the baked cod with steamed asparagus.

Per serving: Calories: 220kcal; Fat: 10g; Carbs: 6g; Protein: 28g; Saturated fat: 2g; Sugar: 3g; Fiber: 3g; Sodium: 70mg

---

| **Stuffed Bell Peppers with Ground Turkey** |

Preparation time: 20 mins

Cooking time: 30 mins

Servings: 4

Ingredients:

• 4 bell peppers, any color, tops and seeds taken out

• 1/2 lb. lean ground turkey

• 1/2 teacup cooked brown rice

• 1/2 teacup low-sodium tomato sauce

• 1/4 teacup cubed onion

• 1/4 teacup cubed tomatoes

• 1/4 teacup low-sodium chicken/vegetable broth

• 1 tsp dried oregano

• Salt and pepper as required

Directions:

1. Warm up oven to 375 deg.F.

2. In a griddle, cook the ground turkey in a middling temp. till it's browned then fully cooked. Drain any extra fat.

3. Inside a container, blend the cooked ground turkey, cooked brown rice, cubed onion, cubed tomatoes, dried oregano, salt, and pepper.

4. Stuff each bell pepper with turkey and rice solution.

5. Place filled peppers in baking dish then pour low-sodium tomato sauce and low-sodium chicken or vegetable broth around them.

6. Cover the baking dish using foil and bake for 25-30 mins or 'til the peppers are soft.

Per serving: Calories: 230kcal; Fat: 6g; Carbs: 23g; Protein: 20g; Saturated fat: 2g; Sugar: 5g; Fiber: 4g; Sodium: 200mg

Snack Time! Little Bites, Big Joy

Snack time is a delightful pause in your day, offering you the opportunity to indulge in little bites of joy. In this chapter, we'll explore a selection of renal diet-friendly snack recipes that are not only delicious but also nourishing. These recipes will keep you and your trusted friend fueled and satisfied among meals.

Crunchy Apple Delight: A Sweet Afternoon Treat

Preparation time: 10 mins

Cooking time: 0 mins

Servings: 2

Ingredients:

- 2 apples, cored and carved
- 2 tbsps almond butter
- 2 tbsps honey
- 2 tbsps severed walnuts (elective for added crunch)
- Cinnamon as required

Directions:

1. Organize the apple slices on a plate.

2. Spray almond butter and honey over the apple slices.

3. Spray the severed walnuts on top for an extra crunch.

4. Dust the dish with cinnamon to include a warm and aromatic flavor.

5. Present your crunchy apple delight instantly and relish this sweet and kidney-friendly treat.

Per serving: Calories: 200kcal; Fat: 10g; Carbs: 25g; Protein: 4g; Saturated fat: 1g; Sugar: 18g; Fiber: 4g; Sodium: 20mg

Variation 1: Pear and Almond Delight

Preparation time: 10 mins

Cooking time: 0 mins

Servings: 2

Ingredients:

- 2 pears, cored and carved
- 2 tbsps almond butter
- 2 tbsps honey
- 2 tbsps carved almonds (elective for added crunch)
- Cinnamon as required

Directions:

1. Follow the same assembly steps as the original recipe, using carved pears instead of apples.

2. Spray almond butter and honey over the pear slices.

3. Spray the carved almonds on top for an extra crunch.

4. Dust the dish with cinnamon to enhance the flavors.

5. Present your delightful pear and almond treat instantly and relish this kidney-friendly variation.

Per serving: Calories: 210kcal; Fat: 11g; Carbs: 27g; Protein: 4g; Saturated fat: 1g; Sugar: 20g; Fiber: 5g; Sodium: 20mg

Variation 2: Banana and Walnut Delight

Preparation time: 10 mins

Cooking time: 0 mins

Servings: 2

Ingredients:

- 2 bananas, carved
- 2 tbsps almond butter
- 2 tbsps honey
- 2 tbsps severed walnuts
- Cinnamon as required

Directions:

1. Follow the same assembly steps as the original recipe, using carved bananas instead of apples.

2. Spray almond butter and honey over the banana slices.

3. Spray the severed walnuts on top for an extra crunch.

4. Dust the dish with cinnamon to amplify the flavors.

5. Present your banana and walnut delight instantly and savor this kidney-friendly twist on the original recipe.

Per serving: Calories: 220kcal; Fat: 11g; Carbs: 30g; Protein: 3g; Saturated fat: 1g; Sugar: 22g; Fiber: 4g; Sodium: 20mg

Nutty Granola Bars: Energy on the Go

Preparation time: 15 mins

Cooking time: 25 mins

Servings: 8

Ingredients:

• 1 teacup old-fashioned oats

• 1/2 teacup mixed nuts (e.g., almonds, walnuts), severed

• 1/2 teacup dried cranberries

• 1/4 teacup honey

• 1/4 teacup almond butter

• 1/2 tsp vanilla extract

• 1/4 tsp salt

Directions:

1. Warm up oven to 350 deg.F. Line an 8x8-inch (20x20 cm) baking pan using parchment paper, leaving some over hang for easy removal.

2. Inside big mixing container, blend the oats, mixed nuts, and dried cranberries.

3. Inside small saucepan, warm the honey, vanilla extract, almond butter, and salt over low heat. Stir till the solution becomes smooth and well blended.

4. Pour the warm honey-almond butter solution over the dry components. Stir till everything is evenly covered.

5. Transfer solution into the prepared baking pan. Press it down firmly with a spatula to create it compact.

6. Bake in to your warmed up oven for 20-25 mins or 'til the edges turn golden brown.

7. Take out from oven then allow it to cool entirely in the pan. Once cooled, lift the parchment paper to take out the granola slab.

8. Cut into 8 bars and store them in an airtight container for an energy-packed, kidney-friendly snack on the go.

Per serving: Calories: 220kcal; Fat: 11g; Carbs: 29g; Protein: 5g; Saturated fat: 1g; Sugar: 15g; Fiber: 4g; Sodium: 75mg

Variation 1: Apricot and Almond Granola Bars

Preparation time: 15 mins

Cooking time: 25 mins

Servings: 8

Ingredients:

• 1 teacup old-fashioned oats

• 1/2 teacup dried apricots, severed

• 1/2 teacup almonds, severed

• 1/4 teacup honey

• 1/4 teacup almond butter

- 1/2 tsp vanilla extract
- 1/4 tsp salt

Directions:

1. Follow the same preparation and baking steps as the original recipe, substituting dried apricots and almonds for dried cranberries and mixed nuts, respectively.

2. Store these apricot and almond granola bars in an airtight container for a kidney-friendly, energy-boosting snack.

Per serving: Calories: 220kcal; Fat: 11g; Carbs: 28g; Protein: 6g; Saturated fat: 1g; Sugar: 15g; Fiber: 4g; Sodium: 75mg

Variation 2: Cherry and Walnut Granola Bars

Preparation time: 15 mins

Cooking time: 25 mins

Servings: 8

Ingredients:

- 1 teacup old-fashioned oats
- 1/2 teacup dried cherries
- 1/2 teacup walnuts, severed
- 1/4 teacup honey
- 1/4 teacup almond butter
- 1/2 tsp vanilla extract
- 1/4 tsp salt

Directions:

1. Follow the same preparation and baking steps as the original recipe, replacing dried cranberries and mixed nuts with dried cherries and severed walnuts, respectively.

2. Store these cherry and walnut granola bars in an airtight container for a kidney-friendly, energy-packed snack option.

Per serving: Calories: 220kcal; Fat: 11g; Carbs: 28g; Protein: 5g; Saturated fat: 1g; Sugar: 15g; Fiber: 4g; Sodium: 75mg

Cool and Creamy Coleslaw: A Refreshing Side

Preparation time: 15 mins

Cooking time: 0 mins

Servings: 4

Ingredients:

- 4 teacups teared up green cabbage
- 1 teacup teared up carrots
- 1/2 teacup plain Greek yogurt
- 2 tbsps mayonnaise
- 1 tbsp apple cider vinegar
- 1 tbsp honey
- 1/2 tsp celery seed (elective)
- Salt and black pepper as required

Directions:

1. Inside big container, blend the teared up cabbage and carrots.

2. Inside a distinct container, whisk collectively the plain Greek yogurt, low-sodium mayonnaise, apple cider vinegar, honey (or sugar substitute), and celery seed if using.

3. Pour creamy dressing over the cabbage and carrot solution. Shake to cover the vegetables evenly.

4. Flavour the coleslaw with salt and black pepper as required.

5. Chill coleslaw in the fridge for 30 mins prior to presenting to allow flavors to meld.

6. Present your cool and creamy coleslaw as a refreshing side dish for a kidney-friendly meal.

Per serving: Calories: 100kcal; Fat: 4g; Carbs: 13g; Protein: 4g; Saturated fat: 1g; Sugar: 8g; Fiber: 3g; Sodium: 150mg

Variation 1: Red Cabbage and Cranberry Slaw

Preparation time: 15 mins

Cooking time: 0 mins

Servings: 4

Ingredients:

• 4 teacups teared up red cabbage

• 1/2 teacup dried cranberries

• 1/2 teacup plain Greek yogurt

• 2 tbsps mayonnaise

• 1 tbsp apple cider vinegar

• 1 tbsp honey

• 1/2 tsp poppy seeds (elective)

• Salt and black pepper as required

Directions:

1. Follow the same preparation and dressing steps as the original recipe, substituting red cabbage for green cabbage and adding dried cranberries for a sweet twist.

2. Chill the red cabbage and cranberry slaw in the fridge as indicated in the main recipe.

3. Present this vibrant and kidney-friendly variation as a refreshing side dish.

Per serving: Calories: 110kcal; Fat: 4g; Carbs: 14g; Protein: 4g; Saturated fat: 1g; Sugar: 10g; Fiber: 3g; Sodium: 150mg

Variation 2: Broccoli and Raisin Coleslaw

Preparation time: 15 mins

Cooking time: 0 mins

Servings: 4

Ingredients:

• 4 teacups teared up broccoli florets

• 1/2 teacup raisins

• 1/2 teacup plain Greek yogurt

• 2 tbsps mayonnaise

• 1 tbsp apple cider vinegar

• 1 tbsp honey

• 1/2 tsp ground mustard (elective)

• Salt and black pepper as required

Directions:

1. Follow the same preparation and dressing steps as the original recipe, using teared up broccoli florets instead of green cabbage and adding raisins for sweetness.

2. Chill the broccoli and raisin coleslaw in the fridge as directed in the main recipe.

3. Present this kidney-friendly variation as a cool and refreshing side dish.

Per serving: Calories: 110kcal; Fat: 4g; Carbs: 14g; Protein: 4g; Saturated fat: 1g; Sugar: 10g; Fiber: 3g; Sodium: 150mg

Fresh Fruit Kabobs with Yogurt Dip

Preparation time: 15 mins

Cooking time: 0 mins

Servings: 2

Ingredients:

• 1 teacup fresh strawberries, hulled and divided

• 1 teacup fresh pineapple chunks

• 1 teacup fresh melon cubes (cantaloupe or honeydew)

- 1/2 teacup low-fat plain Greek yogurt

- 1 tbsp honey (elective, for sweetness)

- 1/2 tsp vanilla extract

Directions:

1. Inside small container, mix Greek yogurt, honey (if using), and vanilla extract to create the yogurt dip.

2. Thread the fresh fruit onto wooden skewers in any order you prefer.

3. Present the fruit kabobs with the yogurt dip on the side.

Per serving: Calories: 150kcal; Fat: 0.5g; Carbs: 33g; Protein: 5g; Saturated fat: 0g; Sugar: 25g; Fiber: 3g; Sodium: 25mg

---

Rice Cake with Almond Butter & Banana Slices

Preparation time: 5 mins

Cooking time: 0 mins

Servings: 1

Ingredients:

- 1 rice cake

- 1 tbsp unsalted almond butter

- 1/2 small banana, finely carved

Directions:

1. Disperse the almond butter evenly over the rice cake.

2. Organize the banana slices on top of the almond butter.

3. Relish your quick and tasty snack!

Per serving: Calories: 200kcal; Fat: 9g; Carbs: 26g; Protein: 4g; Saturated fat: 1g; Sugar: 8g; Fiber: 3g; Sodium: 0mg

Cucumber and Hummus Bites

Preparation time: 10 mins

Cooking time: 0 mins

Servings: 2

Ingredients:

- 1 cucumber, carved into rounds

- 1/2 teacup low-sodium hummus

- Fresh parsley leaves for garnish (elective)

Directions:

1. Organize cucumber slices on a serving plate.

2. Use a small spoon or knife to create a small well in each cucumber slice.

3. Fill each well with a dollop of hummus.

4. Garnish using fresh parsley leaves if anticipated.

5. Present as a healthy and crunchy snack.

Per serving: Calories: 70kcal; Fat: 3g; Carbs: 9g; Protein: 3g; Saturated fat: 0g; Sugar: 2g; Fiber: 2g; Sodium: 150mg

Carrot Sticks with Guacamole

Preparation time: 10 mins

Cooking time: 0 mins

Servings: 2

Ingredients:

- 2 big carrots, that is skinned and cut into sticks

- 1 ripe avocado
- 1 small tomato, cubed
- 1/4 small red onion, finely severed
- 1 piece garlic, crushed
- 1/2 lime, juiced
- Salt and pepper as required

Directions:

1. Inside a container, mash the ripe avocado 'til smooth.

2. Stir in the cubed tomato, severed red onion, salt, crushed garlic, lime juice, and pepper to create the guacamole.

3. Present the carrot sticks with the guacamole for dipping.

Per serving: Calories: 150kcal; Fat: 10g; Carbs: 15g; Protein: 3g; Saturated fat: 1g; Sugar: 4g; Fiber: 7g; Sodium: 80mg

Baked Apple Chips

Preparation time: 10 mins

Cooking time: 2 hrs

Servings: 2

Ingredients:

- 2 big apples, cored and finely carved
- 1/2 tsp ground cinnamon
- Cooking spray

Directions:

1. Warm up oven to 200 deg.F.

2. In container, shake the apple slices with the ground cinnamon to cover them evenly.

3. Line baking sheet using parchment paper and mildly spray it with cooking spray.

4. Organize your apple slices in single layer on baking sheet.

5. Bake in to your warmed up oven for 2 hrs or 'til the apple slices are crisp, turning them halfway through.

6. Let them cool entirely prior to relishing your baked apple chips.

Per serving: Calories: 60kcal; Fat: 0g; Carbs: 15g; Protein: 0g; Saturated fat: 0g; Sugar: 11g; Fiber: 3g; Sodium: 0mg

Homemade Trail Mix with Dried Fruits

Preparation time: 5 mins

Cooking time: 0 mins

Servings: 2

Ingredients:

- 1/2 teacup unsalted almonds
- 1/2 teacup unsalted cashews
- 1/4 teacup dried cranberries
- 1/4 teacup raisins
- 1/4 teacup dried apricots, severed

Directions:

1. Inside a container, blend the unsalted almonds, unsalted cashews, dried cranberries, raisins, and dried apricots.

2. Blend thoroughly and portion into two snack-sized bags for easy grab-and-go.

3. Relish this kidney-friendly trail mix as a satisfying and convenient snack.

Per serving: Calories: 250kcal; Fat: 15g; Carbs: 28g; Protein: 7g; Saturated fat: 1g; Sugar: 17g; Fiber: 4g; Sodium: 0mg

Sip and Savor: Beverages to Brighten Your Day

Beverages can be more than just a source of hydration; they can brighten your day and include a touch of delight to your culinary journey. In this chapter, we'll explore a variety of renal diet-friendly beverage recipes that are not only refreshing but also delicious. These beverages will help you and your trusted friend savor every moment.

Zesty Lemonade: Sunshine in a Glass

Preparation time: 10 mins

Cooking time: 0 mins

Servings: 4

Ingredients:

- 1 teacup freshly squeezed lemon juice
- 4 teacups cold water
- 1/2 teacup honey
- Lemon slices for garnish
- Ice cubes for serving

Directions:

1. In pitcher, blend the freshly squeezed lemon juice, cold water, and honey. Stir well till honey is entirely dissolved.

2. Taste lemonade and adjust the sweetness or tartness by including extra honey or water, if necessary.

3. Chill lemonade in the fridge for almost 30 mins.

4. When ready to present, place ice cubes to glasses then pour the chilled lemonade over the ice.

5. Garnish each glass using a slice of lemon for an extra burst of flavor & visual appeal.

6. Relish your refreshing and kidney-friendly zesty lemonade on a sunny day!

Per serving: Calories: 90kcal; Fat: 0g; Carbs: 25g; Protein: 0g; Saturated fat: 0g; Sugar: 25g; Fiber: 0g; Sodium: 10mg

Variation 1: Raspberry Mint Lemonade

Preparation time: 15 mins

Cooking time: 0 mins

Servings: 4

Ingredients:

- 1 teacup freshly squeezed lemon juice
- 4 teacups cold water
- 1/2 teacup honey
- 1 teacup fresh or frozen raspberries
- Fresh mint leaves for garnish
- Ice cubes for serving

Directions:

1. Follow same preparation steps as the original recipe, adding fresh or frozen raspberries to the lemonade prior to chilling it in the fridge.

2. When serving, include ice cubes to glasses and pour the chilled raspberry mint lemonade over the ice.

3. Garnish each glass using fresh mint leaves for an added refreshing twist.

4. Savor this kidney-friendly variation of zesty lemonade with the delightful combination of raspberries and mint.

Per serving: Calories: 100kcal; Fat: 0g; Carbs: 27g; Protein: 1g; Saturated fat: 0g; Sugar: 26g; Fiber: 2g; Sodium: 10mg

Variation 2: Ginger Lime Lemonade

Preparation time: 15 mins

Cooking time: 0 mins

Servings: 4

Ingredients:

- 1 teacup freshly squeezed lime juice
- 1/2 teacup freshly squeezed lemon juice
- 4 teacups cold water
- 1/2 teacup honey
- 2 tbsps freshly grated ginger

- Lime slices for garnish
- Ice cubes for serving

Directions:

1. Blend the freshly squeezed lime and lemon juice in a pitcher. Include cold water and honey, then stir till the honey is fully dissolved.

2. Mix in the freshly grated ginger and let the flavors infuse for 10 mins.

3. Chill the ginger lime lemonade in the fridge for almost 30 mins.

4. Present over ice cubes, garnishing each glass with a slice of lime for extra tangy and kidney-friendly zesty twist.

Per serving: Calories: 100kcal; Fat: 0g; Carbs: 28g; Protein: 1g; Saturated fat: 0g; Sugar: 27g; Fiber: 0g; Sodium: 10mg

Calming Herbal Teas: Your Relaxation Ritual

Preparation time: 5 mins

Cooking time: 0 mins

Servings: 1

Ingredients:

- 1 tea bag of caffeine-free chamomile tea
- 1 teacup boiling water
- 1 tsp honey (elective)
- 1 slice of lemon (elective)

Directions:

1. Place chamomile tea bag in a teacup.

2. Pour boiling water over the tea bag.

3. Let tea steep for 3-5 mins to allow the chamomile to infuse its calming properties into the water.

4. If desired, place honey to sweeten the tea, or slice of lemon for extra flavor.

5. Sip your chamomile tea slowly and savor the relaxation it brings.

Per serving: Calories: 5kcal; Fat: 0g; Carbs: 2g; Protein: 0g; Saturated fat: 0g; Sugar: 2g; Fiber: 0g; Sodium: 0mg

Variation 1: Lavender and Mint Infusion

Preparation time: 5 mins

Cooking time: 0 mins

Servings: 1

Ingredients:

- 1 tsp dried lavender buds
- 1 tsp dried mint leaves
- 1 teacup boiling water
- 1 tsp honey (elective)

Directions:

1. Put the dried lavender buds and mint leaves in a teapot or infuser.

2. Pour boiling water over the herbs.

3. Let the infusion steep for 3-5 mins to release the calming aromas and flavors.

4. If desired, include honey for a touch of sweetness.

5. Relish your lavender and mint infusion as a soothing alternative to chamomile tea.

Per serving: Calories: 5kcal; Fat: 0g; Carbs: 2g; Protein: 0g; Saturated fat: 0g; Sugar: 2g; Fiber: 0g; Sodium: 0mg

Variation 2: Lemon Balm and Valerian Root Tea

Preparation time: 5 mins

Cooking time: 0 mins

Servings: 1

Ingredients:

- 1 tsp dried lemon balm leaves
- 1 tsp dried valerian root
- 1 teacup boiling water
- 1 tsp honey (elective)

Directions:

1. Blend the dried lemon balm leaves and valerian root in a teapot or infuser.

2. Pour boiling water over the herbs.

3. Allow tea to steep for 5-7 mins to extract the calming properties of lemon balm and valerian.

4. Sweeten with honey if anticipated.

5. Sip your lemon balm and valerian root tea for a soothing and tranquil experience.

Per serving: Calories: 5kcal; Fat: 0g; Carbs: 2g; Protein: 0g; Saturated fat: 0g; Sugar: 2g; Fiber: 0g; Sodium: 0mg

---

Berry Bliss Smoothie: A Sweet Sipper

Preparation time: 5 mins

Cooking time: 0 mins

Servings: 2

Ingredients:

- 1 teacup mixed berries (strawberries, blueberries, raspberries)
- 1 ripe banana
- 1 teacup plain Greek yogurt
- 1/2 teacup unsweetened almond milk
- 1 tbsp honey
- Ice cubes (elective)

Directions:

1. Put the mixed berries, ripe banana, plain Greek yogurt, and almond milk inside a mixer.

2. If desired, include honey or a sugar substitute for sweetness.

3. Blend 'til components are smooth and well blended. If you prefer a thicker texture, include ice cubes and blend again.

4. Pour the berry bliss smoothie into glasses and relish this kidney-friendly sweet sipper.

Per serving: Calories: 150kcal; Fat: 2g; Carbs: 29g; Protein: 8g; Saturated fat: 0g; Sugar: 20g; Fiber: 4g; Sodium: 70mg

Variation 1: Peach and Mango Delight

Preparation time: 5 mins

Cooking time: 0 mins

Servings: 2

Ingredients:

- 1 teacup frozen peaches
- 1/2 teacup frozen mango chunks
- 1 ripe banana
- 1 teacup plain Greek yogurt
- 1/2 teacup unsweetened almond milk
- 1 tbsp honey (elective)
- Ice cubes (elective)

Directions:

1. Follow the same preparation and blending steps as the original recipe, replacing the mixed berries with frozen peaches and mango.

2. Include honey or a sugar substitute for sweetness, if anticipated.

3. Blend 'til smooth and, if needed, include ice cubes for a thicker texture.

4. Present your peach and mango delight for a kidney-friendly twist on the classic smoothie.

Per serving: Calories: 160kcal; Fat: 2g; Carbs: 31g; Protein: 8g; Saturated fat: 0g; Sugar: 24g; Fiber: 3g; Sodium: 70mg

Variation 2: Pineapple and Coconut Dream

Preparation time: 5 mins

Cooking time: 0 mins

Servings: 2

Ingredients:

• 1 teacup frozen pineapple chunks

• 1/2 teacup unsweetened coconut milk

• 1 ripe banana

• 1 teacup plain Greek yogurt

• 1 tbsp honey

• Ice cubes (elective)

Directions:

1. Blend the frozen pineapple chunks, unsweetened coconut milk, ripe banana, and plain Greek yogurt inside a mixer.

2. Sweeten with honey or a sugar substitute if anticipated.

3. Blend 'til the components are smooth and well blended. If you prefer a thicker texture, include ice cubes and blend again.

4. Pour the pineapple and coconut dream smoothie into glasses and relish a tropical, kidney-friendly treat.

Per serving: Calories: 180kcal; Fat: 4g; Carbs: 32g; Protein: 8g; Saturated fat: 3g; Sugar: 22g; Fiber: 3g; Sodium: 80mg

Caffeine-Free Herbal Iced Tea

Preparation time: 5 mins

Cooking time: 10 mins (plus cooling time)

Servings: 4

Ingredients:

• 4 teacups of boiling water

• 4 caffeine-free herbal tea bags (e.g., hibiscus or peppermint)

• 2 tbsps honey (elective, for sweetness)

• Fresh mint leaves (for garnish)

• Ice cubes

Directions:

1. Boil 4 teacups of water then place it over your herbal tea bags in a heatproof pitcher or container.

2. Steep the tea for 5-7 mins. Take out the tea bags.

3. Place honey if anticipated and stir till it dissolves.

4. Let tea cool to room temp., then put in the fridge till it's chilled.

5. Present over ice, garnished using fresh mint leaves.

Per serving: Calories: 15kcal; Fat: 0g; Carbs: 4g; Protein: 0g; Saturated fat: 0g; Sugar: 4g; Fiber: 0g; Sodium: 0mg

Chilled Watermelon Limeade

Preparation time: 10 mins

Cooking time: 0 mins

Servings: 4

Ingredients:

- 3 teacups seedless watermelon, cubed
- 1/4 teacup fresh lime juice
- 1-2 tbsps honey (adjust for sweetness)
- Ice cubes
- Lime slices (for garnish)

Directions:

1. Put the watermelon cubes in blender and blend 'til smooth.

2. Strain watermelon juice through a fine sieve or cheesecloth to take out any solids.

3. In a pitcher, blend the watermelon juice, fresh lime juice, and honey. Stir till well mixed.

4. Chill the solution in the fridge 'til it's cold.

5. Present over ice, garnished with lime slices.

Per serving: Calories: 35kcal; Fat: 0g; Carbs: 9g; Protein: 0g; Saturated fat: 0g; Sugar: 7g; Fiber: 0g; Sodium: 0mg

Cranberry and Pomegranate Spritzer

Preparation time: 5 mins

Cooking time: 0 mins

Servings: 4

Ingredients:

- 1 teacup unsweetened cranberry juice
- 1 teacup unsweetened pomegranate juice
- 2 teacups sparkling water
- Fresh berries (for garnish)
- Ice cubes

Directions:

1. In pitcher, blend the cranberry juice and pomegranate juice.

2. Put the sparkling water then carefully stir to mix.

3. Fill glasses with ice cubes then pour the spritzer over the ice.

4. Garnish using fresh berries, such as raspberries or blueberries.

Per serving: Calories: 35kcal; Fat: 0g; Carbs: 9g; Protein: 0g; Saturated fat: 0g; Sugar: 8g; Fiber: 0g; Sodium: 10mg

Carrot and Ginger Smoothie

Preparation time: 10 mins

Cooking time: 0 mins

Servings: 2

Ingredients:

- 2 big carrots, skinned and severed
- 1-inch piece of fresh ginger, that is skinned and crushed
- 1 teacup unsweetened almond milk
- 1/2 teacup plain Greek yogurt
- 1 tbsp honey (elective, for sweetness)
- Ice cubes

Directions:

1. Put the severed carrots, crushed ginger, almond milk, Greek yogurt, and honey (if using) inside a mixer.

2. Blend 'til the solution is smooth and all the components are well blended.

3. If smoothie is too thick, you can place a little more almond milk to reach consistency.

4. Present in glasses over ice.

Per serving: Calories: 100kcal; Fat: 2g; Carbs: 18g; Protein: 5g; Saturated fat: 0g; Sugar: 12g; Fiber: 3g; Sodium: 70mg

Fresh Orange and Ginger Juice

Preparation time: 5 mins

Cooking time: 0 mins

Servings: 2

Ingredients:

• 4 big oranges, skinned and segmented

• 1-inch piece of fresh ginger, that is skinned and crushed

• Ice cubes (elective)

Directions:

1. Put the orange segments and crushed ginger in a juicer or blender.

2. Blend or juice the components 'til smooth.

3. If you'd like your juice to be colder, you can include ice cubes while blending.

4. Pour into glasses and present instantly.

Per serving: Calories: 80kcal; Fat: 0g; Carbs: 20g; Protein: 2g; Saturated fat: 0g; Sugar: 16g; Fiber: 4g; Sodium: 0mg

Cucumber and Mint Cooler

Preparation time: 10 mins

Cooking time: 0 mins

Servings: 2

Ingredients:

• 1 cucumber, skinned and severed

• 10-12 fresh mint leaves

• 1 lime, juiced

• 2 teacups water

• 1 tbsp honey (elective, for sweetness)

• Ice cubes

Directions:

1. Put the severed cucumber, fresh mint leaves, lime juice, and water inside a mixer.

2. Place honey if you prefer a sweeter taste, and blend 'til smooth.

3. Strain solution through your fine sieve to take out any solid bits.

4. Present the cucumber and mint cooler over ice.

Per serving: Calories: 35kcal; Fat: 0g; Carbs: 9g; Protein: 1g; Saturated fat: 0g; Sugar: 6g; Fiber: 1g; Sodium: 0mg

Sweet Moments: Desserts to Celebrate

Desserts are the perfect way to celebrate life's sweet moments. In this chapter, we'll explore a selection of renal diet-friendly dessert recipes that are not only delicious but also a source of joy. These desserts will include a touch of celebration to your culinary journey, making every meal feel like a special occasion.

Silky Chocolate Pudding: A Spoonful of Happiness

Preparation time: 10 mins

Cooking time: 10 mins

Servings: 4

Ingredients:

- 1/4 teacup unsweetened cocoa powder
- 2 tbsps cornstarch
- 1/4 teacup granulated sugar
- 1/8 tsp salt
- 2 teacups low-potassium milk (e.g., rice milk or almond milk)
- 1/2 tsp vanilla extract
- Whipped cream for garnish (elective)
- Dark chocolate shavings for garnish (elective)

Directions:

1. Inside saucepot, whisk collectively the unsweetened cocoa powder, cornstarch, granulated sugar (or sugar substitute), and salt.

2. Slowly pour in the low-potassium milk while whisking to create a smooth solution.

3. Put the saucepan in a middling temp. then cook the solution, mixing regularly, 'til it thickens. This should take about 8-10 mins.

4. Take saucepan from temp. then stir in the vanilla extract.

5. Pour the chocolate pudding into serving teacups or containers and allow it to cool to room temp.

6. Once cooled, cover each teacup with plastic wrap, ensuring the wrap touches surface of the pudding to prevent a skin from forming.

7. Put in the fridge puddings for almost 2 hrs or 'til they're nicely chilled and set.

8. Before serving, garnish using a dollop of whipped cream and dark chocolate shavings if anticipated.

9. Relish your silky chocolate pudding, a kidney-friendly delight.

Per serving: Calories: 120kcal; Fat: 2g; Carbs: 24g; Protein: 2g; Saturated fat: 1g; Sugar: 14g; Fiber: 2g; Sodium: 80mg

Variation 1: Creamy Banana Chocolate Pudding

Preparation time: 10 mins

Cooking time: 10 mins

Servings: 4

Ingredients:

- 1/4 teacup unsweetened cocoa powder
- 2 tbsps cornstarch
- 1/4 teacup granulated sugar
- 1/8 tsp salt
- 2 teacups low-potassium milk (e.g., rice milk or almond milk)
- 1/2 tsp vanilla extract
- 2 ripe bananas, mashed
- Whipped cream for garnish (elective)

Directions:

1. Follow the same cooking and cooling steps as the original recipe till step 5.

2. After adding the vanilla extract, stir in the mashed ripe bananas to the chocolate pudding.

3. Continue with the chilling and garnishing steps as in the main recipe.

4. Present your creamy banana chocolate pudding, a kidney-friendly variation with a delightful fruit twist.

Per serving: Calories: 130kcal; Fat: 2g; Carbs: 28g; Protein: 2g; Saturated fat: 1g; Sugar: 18g; Fiber: 3g; Sodium: 80mg

Variation 2: Mint Chocolate Pudding

Preparation time: 10 mins

Cooking time: 10 mins

Servings: 4

Ingredients:

- 1/4 teacup unsweetened cocoa powder
- 2 tbsps cornstarch
- 1/4 teacup granulated sugar
- 1/8 tsp salt
- 2 teacups low-potassium milk (e.g., rice milk or almond milk)
- 1/2 tsp mint extract
- Green food coloring (elective)
- Whipped cream for garnish (elective)
- Dark chocolate shavings for garnish (elective)

Directions:

1. Follow the same cooking and cooling steps as the original recipe till step 5.

2. After adding the vanilla extract, stir in the mint extract then green food coloring (if anticipated) to create a mint chocolate flavor and color.

3. Continue with the chilling and garnishing steps as in the main recipe.

4. Present your mint chocolate pudding, a kidney-friendly variation with a refreshing twist.

Per serving: Calories: 120kcal; Fat: 2g; Carbs: 24g; Protein: 2g; Saturated fat: 1g; Sugar: 14g; Fiber: 2g; Sodium: 80mg

Strawberry Sorbet: A Cool Treat for Warm Days

Preparation time: 10 mins

Cooking time: 0 mins

Servings: 4

Ingredients:

- 1 lb. fresh strawberries, hulled and divided
- 1/2 teacup granulated sugar
- 2 tbsps lemon juice
- 1/4 teacup water
- Fresh mint leaves for garnish (elective)

Directions:

1. Inside a mixer, blend the fresh strawberries, granulated sugar (or sugar substitute), lemon juice, and water.

2. Blend till the solution is smooth and the sugar is entirely dissolved.

3. Pour strawberry solution into a shallow container and cover it with plastic wrap.

4. Freeze for 4-6 hrs, or 'til the sorbet is firm, stirring every 30 mins to prevent ice crystals from forming.

5. When ready to present, let sorbet sit at room temp. for a couple of mins to soften mildly.

6. Scoop the strawberry sorbet into containers or teacups, garnish using fresh mint leaves if anticipated, and relish this refreshing kidney-friendly treat.

Per serving: Calories: 110kcal; Fat: 0g; Carbs: 28g; Protein: 1g; Saturated fat: 0g; Sugar: 26g; Fiber: 2g; Sodium: 0mg

Variation 1: Raspberry Delight Sorbet

Preparation time: 10 mins

Cooking time: 0 mins

Servings: 4

Ingredients:

- 1 lb. fresh raspberries
- 1/2 teacup granulated sugar
- 2 tbsps lemon juice
- 1/4 teacup water
- Fresh mint leaves for garnish (elective)

Directions:

1. Follow the same preparation and freezing steps as the original recipe, substituting fresh raspberries for strawberries to create a delightful raspberry sorbet.

2. Garnish using fresh mint leaves for added appeal and flavor.

3. Relish your raspberry delight sorbet as a kidney-friendly alternative.

Per serving: Calories: 110kcal; Fat: 0g; Carbs: 28g; Protein: 1g; Saturated fat: 0g; Sugar: 26g; Fiber: 8g; Sodium: 0mg

Variation 2: Mango Tango Sorbet

Preparation time: 10 mins

Cooking time: 0 mins

Servings: 4

Ingredients:

- 1 lb. fresh mango chunks (or use frozen mango chunks for convenience)
- 1/2 teacup granulated sugar
- 2 tbsps lime juice
- 1/4 teacup water
- Fresh mint leaves for garnish (elective)

Directions:

1. Follow the same preparation and freezing steps as the original recipe, using fresh or frozen mango chunks to create a tropical mango sorbet.

2. Garnish using fresh mint leaves for a touch of freshness.

3. Savor your mango tango sorbet as a kidney-friendly alternative to strawberry sorbet.

Per serving: Calories: 120kcal; Fat: 0g; Carbs: 31g; Protein: 1g; Saturated fat: 0g; Sugar: 29g; Fiber: 2g; Sodium: 0mg

Heavenly Pound Cake: A Slice of Joy

Preparation time: 20 mins

Cooking time: 1 hr

Servings: 12

Ingredients:

- 1 teacup unsalted butter, softened
- 2 teacups granulated sugar
- 4 big eggs
- 2 teacups all-purpose flour
- 1/2 tsp salt
- 1/2 teacup low-potassium milk (e.g., rice milk or almond milk)
- 1 tsp vanilla extract
- Zest of one lemon
- Powdered sugar for dusting (elective)

Directions:

1. Warm up oven to 325 deg.F. Grease and flour a 9x5-inch (23x13 cm) loaf pan.

2. Inside big mixing container, cream the softened unsalted butter and granulated sugar (or sugar substitute) 'til light and fluffy.

3. Put the eggs one at a time, mixing well after each addition.

4. Inside a distinct container, blend the all-purpose flour and salt.

5. Slowly place dry components to the butter solution, alternating with the low-potassium milk, starting and ending with the flour solution.

6. Stir in vanilla extract and lemon zest.

7. Pour batter in to your prepared loaf pan and smooth the top.

8. Bake for 60-70 mins, or 'til a toothpick immersed into the center comes out clean.

9. Allow lb. cake cool in pan for 10 mins, then take out it from the pan then place it on your wire stand to cool entirely.

10. Dust with powdered sugar, if anticipated.

11. Slice and present your heavenly lb. cake for a kidney-friendly dessert or snack.

Per serving: Calories: 300kcal; Fat: 14g; Carbs: 40g; Protein: 4g; Saturated fat: 8g; Sugar: 24g; Fiber: 1g; Sodium: 100mg

Variation 1: Orange Almond Pound Cake
Preparation time: 20 mins

Cooking time: 1 hr

Servings: 12

Ingredients:

- 1 teacup unsalted butter, softened

- 2 teacups granulated sugar

- 4 big eggs

- 2 teacups all-purpose flour

- 1/2 tsp salt

- 1/2 teacup low-potassium milk (e.g., rice milk or almond milk)

- 1 tsp almond extract

- Zest of one orange

- Powdered sugar for dusting (elective)

Directions:

1. Follow the same preparation and baking steps as the original recipe, with the following modifications:

2. Replace lemon zest using the zest of one orange.

3. Stir in 1 tsp of almond extract in addition to the vanilla extract.

4. Dust with powdered sugar as an elective finishing touch.

5. Present your orange almond lb. cake as a kidney-friendly twist on the classic.

Per serving: Calories: 300kcal; Fat: 14g; Carbs: 40g; Protein: 4g; Saturated fat: 8g; Sugar: 24g; Fiber: 1g; Sodium: 100mg

Variation 2: Lemon Blueberry Pound Cake
Preparation time: 20 mins

Cooking time: 1 hr

Servings: 12

Ingredients:

- 1 teacup unsalted butter, softened

- 2 teacups granulated sugar

- 4 big eggs

- 2 teacups all-purpose flour
- 1/2 tsp salt
- 1/2 teacup low-potassium milk (e.g., rice milk or almond milk)
- 1 tsp vanilla extract
- Zest of one lemon
- 1 teacup fresh or frozen low-potassium blueberries
- Powdered sugar for dusting (elective)

Directions:

1. Follow the same preparation and baking steps as the original recipe, with the following modifications:

2. Replace lemon zest using the zest of one lemon.

3. Wrap in 1 teacup of your fresh or frozen low-potassium blueberries into the batter prior to pouring it into the loaf pan.

4. Dust with powdered sugar as an elective finishing touch.

5. Present your lemon blueberry lb. cake as a kidney-friendly variation with a burst of fruity flavor.

Per serving: Calories: 310kcal; Fat: 14g; Carbs: 42g; Protein: 4g; Saturated fat: 8g; Sugar: 26g; Fiber: 1g; Sodium: 100mg

Baked Apples with Cinnamon and Nutmeg

Preparation time: 10 mins

Cooking time: 30 mins

Servings: 2

Ingredients:

- 2 medium-sized apples
- 1/2 tsp ground cinnamon
- 1/4 tsp ground nutmeg
- 1/2 teacup water
- 1 tbsp honey

Directions:

1. Warm up oven to 375 deg.F.

2. Wash and core the apples, removing the seeds and leaving the skin on.

3. Inside small container, mix the cinnamon and nutmeg.

4. Put the apples in a baking dish and spray the cinnamon and nutmeg solution over them.

5. Pour the water into the bottom of the baking dish.

6. If desired, spray honey over the apples for a touch of sweetness (in moderation).

7. Cover the baking dish using foil then bake for 30 mins or 'til the apples are soft.

8. Present the baked apples warm, with a spoonful of the cooking liquid if anticipated.

Per serving: Calories: 80kcal; Fat: 0.3g; Carbs: 21g; Protein: 0.4g; Saturated fat: 0g; Sugar: 17g; Fiber: 4g; Sodium: 2mg

Chia Seed Pudding with Fresh Berries

Preparation time: 5 mins (plus refrigeration time)

Cooking time: 0 mins

Servings: 2

Ingredients:

- 2 tbsps chia seeds
- 1 teacup unsweetened almond milk

- 1/2 tsp vanilla extract
- 1 teacup mixed fresh berries (e.g., strawberries, blueberries, raspberries)
- 1 tbsp honey

Directions:

1. In container, blend the chia seeds, almond milk, and vanilla extract. Stir well.

2. Put in the fridge solution for 2 hrs or overnight to allow chia seeds to absorb liquid and thicken.

3. Before serving, stir the chia pudding to ensure an even consistency.

4. Present the chia pudding in containers, topped with fresh mixed berries and a spray of honey (elective, in moderation).

Per serving: Calories: 150kcal; Fat: 5g; Carbs: 23g; Protein: 4g; Saturated fat: 0.5g; Sugar: 10g; Fiber: 11g; Sodium: 80mg

---

Poached Pears in Ginger Syrup

Preparation time: 10 mins

Cooking time: 20 mins

Servings: 2

Ingredients:

- 2 ripe but firm pears
- 2 teacups water
- 1-inch piece of fresh ginger, that is skinned and carved
- 1 cinnamon stick
- 2-3 pieces (elective)
- 2 tbsps honey

Directions:

1. Peel the pears and leave them whole, with the stem intact if possible.

2. Inside saucepot, blend the water, ginger, cinnamon stick, and pieces (if using).

3. Simmer the solution, then include the pears.

4. Cover the saucepan and let the pears simmer for 15-20 mins, or 'til they are soft but not mushy.

5. Take out the pears and set them aside.

6. Continue to simmer the ginger syrup till it reduces and thickens mildly.

7. If desired, spray honey over the poached pears (elective, in moderation).

8. Present the poached pears drizzled with the ginger syrup.

Per serving: Calories: 120kcal; Fat: 0.2g; Carbs: 32g; Protein: 1g; Saturated fat: 0g; Sugar: 21g; Fiber: 5g; Sodium: 5mg

---

Frozen Yogurt with Mango Puree

Preparation time: 5 mins

Cooking time: 0 mins (plus freezing time)

Servings: 2

Ingredients:

- 1 teacup plain low-fat or non-fat yogurt (low in phosphorus)
- 1 teacup frozen mango chunks (unsweetened)
- 2 tbsps honey

Directions:

1. Inside a mixer, blend the plain yogurt and frozen mango chunks.

2. Blend till you have a smooth and creamy solution.

3. If desired, spray honey over the frozen yogurt (elective, in moderation).

4. Present instantly as a refreshing dessert.

Per serving: Calories: 120kcal; Fat: 0.2g; Carbs: 29g; Protein: 3g; Saturated fat: 0g; Sugar: 27g; Fiber: 2g; Sodium: 45mg

Rice Pudding with Raisins and Cinnamon

Preparation time: 5 mins

Cooking time: 25 mins

Servings: 2

Ingredients:

• 1/2 teacup white rice (washed well)

• 2 teacups unsweetened almond milk

• 2 tbsps raisins

• 1/2 tsp ground cinnamon

• 1 tbsp honey

Directions:

1. Inside saucepot, blend the washed white rice and unsweetened almond milk.

2. Simmer the solution, then decrease the temp. to low, cover, then cook for 20-25 mins, mixing irregularly, 'til the rice is soft then the solution thickens.

3. Stir in the raisins and ground cinnamon.

4. If desired, spray honey over the rice pudding (elective, in moderation).

5. Present the rice pudding warm or chilled.

Per serving: Calories: 190kcal; Fat: 1.5g; Carbs: 43g; Protein: 2.5g; Saturated fat: 0g; Sugar: 10g; Fiber: 1g; Sodium: 160mg

Grilled Pineapple with Honey Drizzle

Preparation time: 10 mins

Cooking time: 5 mins

Servings: 2

Ingredients:

• 1 small pineapple, skinned and cored, and cut into rings

• 1 tbsp honey

Directions:

1. Warm up grill or your stovetop grill pan to med-high temp.

2. Grill your pineapple rings for around 2-3 mins on all sides, or 'til they have grill marks and are fully heated.

3. Take out the grilled pineapple rings from the grill.

4. If desired, spray honey over the grilled pineapple (elective, in moderation).

5. Present the grilled pineapple as a simple and delicious dessert.

Per serving: Calories: 70kcal; Fat: 0.2g; Carbs: 19g; Protein: 0.6g; Saturated fat: 0g; Sugar: 13g; Fiber: 2g; Sodium: 0mg

Navigating Your Diet with Grace

Successfully following a renal diet is not just about the recipes and meals you prepare at home; it's also about how you navigate your diet gracefully in various situations. Here, we'll explore tips and guidance to help you manage your renal diet with ease and confidence.

Fluids: Finding Your Perfect Balance

Balancing your fluid intake is a fundamental aspect of the renal diet. It's essential for managing your kidney health and maintaining overall well-being. Here are three valuable tips to help you find the perfect fluid balance:

1. **Monitor and Track:** Keeping a fluid intake journal can be a game-changer. Record every glass of water, teacup of tea, and container of soup you consume. This will not only help you stay within your recommended fluid limit but also provide valuable insights into your hydration habits.

2. **Choose the Right Beverages:** Opt for beverages that not only quench your thirst but also contribute to your overall well-being. Herbal teas, diluted fruit juices, and water-rich fruits like watermelon are excellent choices. Experiment with different flavors and textures to keep your hydration routine exciting.

3. **Set a Schedule:** Establish a routine for your fluid intake. This can help regulate your hydration and make it easier to manage. For example, you might decide to drink a glass of water at specific times throughout the day. Consistency can be your best ally in maintaining the right fluid balance.

Dining Out: Enjoying Meals with Friends, Stress-Free

Dining out can be a delightful experience, even with dietary restrictions. With a couple of thoughtful strategies, you can savor meals with friends and family while staying on track with your renal diet. Here are three tips to help you dine out stress-free:

1. **Research and Plan Ahead:** Before heading to a restaurant, look up the menu online if available. Most restaurants provide their menus on their websites. This allows you to identify kidney-friendly options and plan your order in advance.

2. **Customize Your Order:** Don't hesitate to request modifications to your dish. Ask for sauces or dressings on the side, request grilled or steamed preparations instead of fried, and substitute high-potassium sides with renal-friendly alternatives like a baked potato without the skin.

3. **Communicate with Your Server:** When you arrive at the restaurant, inform your server about your dietary restrictions. They can communicate your needs to the kitchen staff and ensure your meal aligns with your renal diet. Don't be shy about specifying your requirements; it's essential for your health.

Potassium and Phosphorus: Making Sense of It All

Potassium and phosphorus are two crucial minerals to manage on a renal diet. Understanding their sources and how to balance them is key to maintaining kidney health. Here are three tips to help you make sense of potassium and phosphorus:

1. **Know High-Potassium Foods:** Familiarize yourself with foods that are high in potassium, such as bananas, oranges, and potatoes. While these are nutritious, they should be consumed in moderation. It's not about avoiding them entirely but being mindful of your portions.

2. **Low-Potassium Alternatives:** Explore low-potassium alternatives to your favorite high-potassium foods. For instance, replace potatoes with cauliflower or sweet potatoes, or swap out oranges for apples or berries.

3. **Phosphorus Management:** High-phosphorus foods can be challenging to control, especially with processed foods. Read labels diligently and select products that are lower in phosphorus. Fresh, unprocessed foods are generally lower in phosphorus content, making them a safer bet.

By implementing these tips, you can navigate your renal diet with grace and confidence. Finding your fluid balance, dining out without stress, and managing potassium and phosphorus will become second nature as you continue on your culinary adventure. Remember, with patience and dedication, you can maintain a balanced and delicious diet that supports your kidney health and overall well-being.

You're Not Alone: Emotional Support and Tips

Living with the dietary restrictions of a renal diet can be challenging, both physically and emotionally. It's essential to acknowledge and address the emotional aspects of managing a chronic health condition. Here, we'll explore how to embrace the ups and downs, stay positive, and connect with others for support on your journey.

Embracing the Ups and Downs: It's Okay to Feel

Living with a renal diet can bring about a range of emotions, from frustration to determination and everything in between. It's crucial to acknowledge these feelings and give yourself the space to experience them fully. Here are some tips for embracing the emotional ups and downs:

1. **Practice Mindfulness:** Take time each day to be present in the moment. Mindfulness practices such as meditation, deep breathing, or gentle yoga can help you acknowledge your emotions without judgment.

2. **Keep a Journal:** Engaging in the act of putting your thoughts and feelings on paper can offer a profound sense of release and clarity. Utilize your journal as a means to articulate not only your challenges and successes but also everything in between. This invaluable tool can aid in reflection and the processing of your emotions.

3. **Seek Professional Help:** Should you encounter difficulties in handling your emotions while navigating the challenges of a renal diet, it's advisable to connect with a mental health expert. Seeking therapy can offer a secure environment for delving into your emotions and crafting effective coping strategies specific to your dietary journey.

Staying Positive: Little Tips for Big Smiles

Sustaining a positive outlook is crucial for one's holistic well-being. While living with dietary restrictions may present challenges, it's essential to find joy in the small things and stay optimistic. Here are some tips to help you cultivate a positive outlook:

1. **Practice Gratitude:** Take a moment each day to reflect on the things you are grateful for. Whether it's a supportive friend, a delicious meal, or a beautiful sunset, cultivating gratitude can shift your focus towards the positives in your life.

2. **Engage in Hobbies:** Dedicate time to activities that bring you joy and fulfillment. Whether it's gardening, painting, or playing a musical instrument, engaging in hobbies can provide a sense of accomplishment and happiness.

3. **Celebrate Small Victories:** Acknowledge and celebrate every accomplishment, no matter how small. Whether it's trying a new kidney-friendly recipe or adhering to your fluid intake goals, recognizing your achievements can boost your self-esteem and motivation.

Finding Your Tribe: Connecting with Fellow Warriors

Connecting with others who understand the challenges of a renal diet can provide a sense of camaraderie and support. Building a community of individuals who share similar experiences can offer empathy, encouragement, and valuable insights. Here are some ways to find your tribe:

1. **Join Support Groups:** Look for local or online support groups for individuals living with kidney conditions. These groups can provide a platform for sharing experiences, seeking advice, and offering emotional support.

2. **Attend Wellness Events:** Participate in wellness events, workshops, or seminars focused on kidney health. These gatherings provide opportunities to connect with healthcare professionals, learn about the latest research, and meet others on a similar journey.

3. **Utilize Online Forums:** Explore online forums and communities dedicated to renal health and dietary management. Engaging in discussions, asking questions, and sharing your experiences can create a sense of belonging and provide valuable insights from peers.

Remember, you are not alone on this journey. Embracing your emotions, cultivating a positive mindset, and connecting with others who understand your experiences can provide the emotional support and encouragement you need to thrive on your renal diet. Through shared experiences and mutual support, you can navigate the challenges with strength and resilience.

Your Questions, Answered

Here, we'll address 10 common queries about the renal diet, aiming to provide clear and informative answers to some of the most frequently asked questions. Let's dive in and clear things up!

10 common Queries: Let's Clear Things Up!

How can I make my meals more flavorful without using salt?

You can include flavor to your dishes by using herbs, spices, and salt-free seasoning blends. Ingredients like garlic, onion, lemon, and vinegar can also enhance the taste of your meals without relying on salt.

Can I still enjoy sweets on a renal diet?

Yes, you can relish sweets in moderation. Consider using kidney-friendly sweeteners like stevia or erythritol and exploring recipes that use low-phosphorus components for desserts.

What are some good protein sources for a renal diet?

Lean protein sources like poultry, fish, egg whites, and tofu are excellent choices. Be mindful of portion sizes to avoid overloading on protein.

Is it okay to drink alcohol on a renal diet?

Moderate alcohol consumption may be acceptable for some individuals with kidney disease, but it's essential to consult with your healthcare provider. Alcohol can interact with medications and affect kidney function, so it's best to get personalized guidance.

How can I manage my fluid intake without feeling thirsty all the time?

Chewing gum, sucking on ice chips, and using a moist cloth to wet your mouth can help alleviate the feeling of thirst. Staying cool and avoiding salty foods can also reduce thirst.

Can I eat dairy products on a renal diet?

Dairy products are a source of calcium and protein, but they can also be high in phosphorus. Choose low-phosphorus options like almond milk or limit your intake of dairy products.

How can I manage my phosphorus intake effectively?

Read food labels to identify phosphorus content and choose lower-phosphorus products. Focus on fresh and unprocessed foods, as they tend to be lower in phosphorus.

Are there any kidney-friendly fast-food options?

Some fast-food restaurants offer healthier choices, like grilled chicken or salads. Avoiding high-sodium condiments and choosing water or a kidney-friendly beverage can also make fast-food options more suitable for a renal diet.

Can I use salt substitutes on a renal diet?

Salt substitutes often contain potassium, which can be problematic for individuals with kidney disease. Consult with your healthcare provider prior to using salt substitutes, and consider potassium-free seasoning alternatives.

How often should I get my kidney function checked?

The frequency of kidney function tests will vary depending on your individual health and the stage of your kidney disease. Your healthcare provider will determine the appropriate schedule for monitoring your kidney function, which may include blood tests and urine tests.

By addressing these common questions, we hope to provide you with a better understanding of the renal diet and how to navigate it successfully. Remember that personalized guidance from a healthcare provider or renal dietitian is crucial, as dietary recommendations can vary based on your specific health needs and circumstances.

Continuing the Journey Hand in Hand

As you've journeyed through this renal diet cookbook, you've learned about the principles of the renal diet, discovered a range of delicious recipes, and gained insights into the emotional and practical aspects of managing your kidney health. Now, it's time to look to the future and continue this adventure, hand in hand with your loved ones.

Embracing Tomorrow: The Adventure Continues

Sharing the Culinary Experience

One of the joys of cooking is sharing your creations with friends and family. It's an opportunity to connect, bond, and savor the delicious results of your culinary adventures together. While the renal diet may have its challenges, it can also be an avenue for culinary creativity and shared experiences.

To continue the journey, we encourage you to create your own kidney-friendly recipes that you can relish with your loved ones. Get your trusted friend involved, set a date, and embark on a new culinary adventure together. Here are some tips to get you started:

1. **Plan a Cooking Date:** Choose a day and time that works for both you and your cooking companion. It could be a weekend afternoon or an evening when you both have some free time.

2. **Select Your Recipes:** Decide on a couple of renal-friendly recipes you'd like to prepare together. It could be a complete meal or just a dish or two, depending on your preferences.

3. **Shop Together:** Head to the grocery store or shop online for the components you need. Make a shopping list to ensure you have everything on hand when you start cooking.

4. **Divide and Conquer:** Assign tasks to each person. One can focus on chopping and preparing components, while the other can handle the cooking. This way, you'll work as a team to create your meal.

5. **Share the Experience:** While you're cooking, take the time to share stories, catch up on each other's lives, and relish the process. Cooking together can be a fun and bonding experience.

6. **Taste and Adjust:** Once your meal is ready, taste it together and make any necessary adjustments to the seasoning or presentation. Your collective efforts will result in a delicious and kidney-friendly dish.

7. **Savor the Meal:** Sit down and savor the meal you've prepared. Appreciate the effort you both put into creating something tasty and healthy.

Creating Your Own Recipes

Beyond cooking the recipes in this cookbook, you can also experiment and create your own kidney-friendly dishes. Here's how to get started:

1. **Understand Renal Diet Principles:** Familiarize yourself with the key principles of the renal diet, including managing sodium, potassium, phosphorus, protein, and fluid intake. This knowledge will guide your recipe creation.

2. **Start with Familiar Ingredients:** Begin with components you know are safe for a renal diet, such as lean meats, low-potassium vegetables, and fresh herbs.

3. **Combine Flavors and Textures:** Experiment with different flavor combinations and textures to create interesting and delicious dishes. For example, try pairing a tangy vinaigrette with a crunchy salad or marinating lean protein in kidney-friendly herbs and spices.

4. **Use Online Resources:** There are many online resources and renal diet cookbooks that offer creative renal-friendly recipes. You can draw inspiration from them and adapt the recipes to your preferences.

5. **Keep a Recipe Journal:** As you experiment with new recipes, keep a journal of your creations. Note the components and quantities you used, as well as any adjustments for the next time.

6. **Seek Feedback:** Share your dishes with friends and family and ask for their feedback. Their input can help you refine your recipes and make them even better.

The Culinary Journey Continues

Just as the adventure doesn't end with the final page of this cookbook, your dietary journey is unique and ever-evolving. With every meal you prepare, every dish you create, and every moment you share with friends and family, you embark on a culinary exploration guided by the renal diet. While this path may present its challenges, it also offers an exciting opportunity to strengthen connections with your loved ones.

As you continue your journey, it's essential to remember that everyone's needs can be a bit different. Your trusted friend, the support of your loved ones, and the knowledge you've gained will be with you every step of the way. So, just like you embrace tomorrow with open arms and continue exploring new recipes, remember to consult with a nutritionist or doctor about your specific dietary needs. This way, you can relish the flavors and experiences that lie ahead, ensuring a bright and flavorful future on your renal diet adventure!

Glossary of Terms

To ensure that every term used in this guide is clear and friendly, here's a glossary to help you understand the language and terminology.

Unraveling the Language: Making Every Term Clear and Friendly

Antioxidants: Compounds that combat free radicals and oxidative stress, found in colorful fruits and vegetables.

B Vitamins: A group of vitamins that support various bodily functions, including energy metabolism and muscle health, often obtained from sources like whole grains, lean meats, and eggs.

Baking Sheets and Pans: Cookware for baking, used in preparing sweet and savory dishes.

Blender or Food Processor: Appliances used for pureeing, blending, and creating smooth textures in dishes and beverages.

Calcium: A mineral important for bone health, with low-phosphorus alternatives like almond milk recommended in the renal diet.

Calorie Intake: The number of calories consumed through food and beverages, which provides the body with energy for daily activities.

Can Opener: A tool for opening tinned components, such as low-sodium beans and vegetables.

Canned Beans: Canned beans that are low in sodium and can present as a source of plant-based protein.

Canned Low-Potassium Fruits: Canned fruits that are low in potassium, like peaches and pears.

Canned Low-Potassium Vegetables: Canned vegetables that are low in potassium, such as green beans and carrots.

Colander: A kitchen tool for draining liquids from foods, like rinsing fruits and vegetables or draining pasta.

Cooking Oils: Kidney-friendly cooking oils like olive oil, canola oil, and grapeseed oil.

Cutting Boards: Kitchen tools for chopping and preparing components, with separate boards for meats and fruits/vegetables to prevent cross-contamination.

Dietary Regimen: A structured plan for food and nutrition, often used to manage health conditions or meet specific dietary goals.

Dried Herbs and Spices: Flavor-enhancing components for recipes, used to include taste without relying on salt.

Electrolyte Balance: The equilibrium of electrolytes, such as sodium, potassium, and phosphorus, in the body, crucial for maintaining proper muscle and nerve function, among other physiological processes.

Fluid Intake: Monitoring the consumption of liquids, including water and beverages, to maintain fluid balance, prevent swelling, and manage high blood pressure in kidney disease.

Fluid Retention: The accumulation of extra fluid in the body, often causing swelling, a common issue in kidney disease.

Fluid Retention: The accumulation of extra fluids in the body, often associated with kidney disease, leading to swelling (edema) and increased blood pressure.

Flour Alternatives: Kidney-friendly flour alternatives like almond flour or coconut flour for baking.

Food Allergen Warnings: Notifications on food labels that alert consumers to the presence of common allergens in the product.

Food Labels: Information on packaging that provides details about the nutrient content of a product, including sodium, potassium, phosphorus, protein, and serving size.

Fresh Produce: Unprocessed fruits and vegetables, often recommended in the renal diet for lower potassium content.

Garlic Press: A tool for quickly and simply mincing garlic.

Gratitude: A practice of acknowledging and appreciating the positive aspects of life and experiences.

Grater and Zester: Tools for grating components like citrus zest or cheese for flavor enhancement.

Gravitation: A low-sodium or salt-free option, commonly used to indicate reduced sodium content in foods.

High Blood Pressure: Elevated blood pressure, which can lead to various health problems, including cardiovascular issues and kidney complications.

Herbal Teas: Infusions made from herbs, spices, flowers, or other plant materials, often caffeine-free and consumed for their flavor and potential health benefits.

Homeostasis: Refers to the ability of the body or a cell to seek and maintain a condition of internal stability, such as the balance of electrolytes, fluids, and other physiological processes, for optimal functioning.

Hydrator: A beverage or food item that helps maintain or improve hydration.

Iron: A mineral essential for preventing anemia, which can be addressed through lean cuts of meat, poultry, and fish along with vitamin C-rich foods.

Knives: Essential kitchen tools for cutting, including chef's knives, paring knives, and serrated knives.

Low-Phosphorus Cereals: Breakfast cereals low in both phosphorus and potassium.

Low-Phosphorus Snacks: Snack options low in phosphorus for those in-between meal munchies.

Low-Sodium Broth: A versatile ingredient for soups and stews, available in low-sodium or no-salt-added versions.

Low-Sodium Condiments: Condiments with reduced sodium content, including low-sodium soy sauce, ketchup, and salt-free herb and spice blends.

Low-Phosphorus Cereals: Breakfast cereals low in both phosphorus and potassium.

Low-Phosphorus Snacks: Snack options low in phosphorus for those in-between meal munchies.

Low-Sodium Condiments: Condiments with reduced sodium content, including low-sodium soy sauce, ketchup, and salt-free herb and spice blends.

Low-Sodium Diet: A specialized dietary plan that restricts the intake of salt, often recommended for individuals with high blood pressure or kidney disease.

Measuring Cups and Spoons: Tools for precise measurement of components in recipes.

Mindful Eating: A practice of being present and fully engaged in the eating experience, paying close attention to the sensory aspects of food and one's body's cues.

Mindfulness: A state of being fully present and engaged in the moment, often achieved through meditation and deep breathing exercises.

Mixing Bowls: Containers of various sizes used for mixing components and preparing dishes.

Nuts and Seeds: Kidney-friendly nuts and seeds such as almonds, cashews, and chia seeds for added texture and flavor in dishes.

Nutrients: Substances in food that provide nourishment and support various bodily functions, including fiber, calcium, iron, vitamin D, B vitamins, and antioxidants.

Oven Mitts: Protective gear for handling hot dishes and cookware.

Phosphorus: A mineral that, when consumed in extra, can weaken bones and contribute to heart problems, making it important to monitor in the renal diet.

Pots and Pans: Cookware for various cooking techniques, including non-stick frying pans, saucepans, stockpots, and sauté pans.

Protein: An essential nutrient for overall health, but excessive protein intake can strain the kidneys, necessitating careful balance in the renal diet.

Protein Metabolism: The process by which the body breaks down and uses proteins for various functions, and the elimination of waste products, particularly urea, from protein metabolism.

Renal Diet: A specialized dietary plan designed to support kidney function and manage kidney-related health issues by controlling the intake of specific nutrients like sodium, potassium, phosphorus, and protein.

Rice and Pasta: Kidney-friendly grains for a variety of recipes, such as white rice and pasta.

Storage Containers: Airtight containers for storing leftovers and prepared components.

Support Groups: Communities of individuals with shared experiences who come together to offer emotional support, share information, and provide encouragement to one another.

Sugar Alternatives: Kidney-friendly sugar substitutes like stevia or erythritol for sweetening recipes.

Sodium: A mineral found in salt that, when consumed in extra, can lead to fluid retention and increased blood pressure, making it a key concern in the renal diet.

Thermometer: A tool for measuring the internal temp. of foods, ensuring safe and proper cooking.

Toxin Accumulation: The buildup of waste products and toxins in the body due to impaired kidney function, often leading to a condition called uremia.

Uremia: A condition associated with kidney failure where waste products are retained in the blood, leading to symptoms like nausea, vomiting, fatigue, and loss of appetite.

Utensils: Kitchen tools such as spatulas, tongs, whisks, and ladles for various culinary tasks.

Vinegar: Flavorful additives like balsamic vinegar or rice vinegar that include a tangy punch to meals.

Vitamin D: A vitamin important for bone health, which may require supplements in cases of compromised kidney function.

A Heartfelt Note

Gratitude and Warmth: For Sharing This Culinary Journey

As we reach the final page of this renal diet cookbook, it's with a heart full of gratitude and warmth that we extend our appreciation to you, our dear reader. Your dedication to exploring this culinary adventure and your commitment to managing your kidney health inspire us beyond words.

The journey through a renal diet can be challenging, marked by dietary restrictions and the need for careful meal planning. Yet, within this challenge lies a world of opportunity, creativity, and connection. It's a journey that you've undertaken with determination and grace, and for that, we commend you.

Throughout this cookbook, we've aimed to provide you with not just recipes but a wealth of knowledge, tips, and insights to create your renal diet journey more manageable and enjoyable.

We've walked hand in hand with you through the basics of the renal diet, equipped you with essential kitchen tools, and guided you in making smart dietary choices.

We've also ventured into the emotional aspects of living with dietary restrictions, offering support and encouragement for the ups and downs you may encounter. You're not alone on this path, and we hope you've found solace in the words and advice provided.

Our wish is that you've not only discovered delicious and kidney-friendly recipes but also experienced the joys of sharing meals with loved ones. Cooking can be a profoundly connecting experience, and we encourage you to continue to embrace the culinary journey with open arms and an adventurous spirit.

Your trusted friend and fellow culinary explorer, whether that's a family member, a dear friend, or a partner, has been there every step of the way, making this journey richer and more meaningful. The bonds you've strengthened through shared meals are to be cherished.

As you move forward, we encourage you to keep the culinary adventure alive. Create your own kidney-friendly recipes, explore new flavors, and savor every moment shared around the table. Embrace tomorrow with optimism and a zest for the culinary wonders that await.

We hope this cookbook has been a valuable resource on your renal diet journey. Always remember that you have the knowledge, the support, and the determination to manage your kidney health with grace and resilience. You are the hero of your story, and we believe in your ability to craft a bright and flavorful future.

INDEX

Mexican-Inspired Black Bean and Corn Salad; 72

Mint Chocolate Pudding; 56

Nutty Granola Bars; 43

Oatmeal with Fresh Berries; 21

Orange Almond Pound Cake; 58

Peach and Almond Oatmeal; 17

Peach and Mango Delight; 51

Pear and Almond Delight; 42

Personalized Quinoa Salad Bowls; 69

Pineapple and Coconut Dream; 52

Poached Egg on Whole Grain Toast; 22

Poached Pears in Ginger Syrup; 60

Quinoa and Black Bean Bowl; 30

Quinoa Breakfast Bowl; 21

Raspberry Delight Sorbet; 57

Raspberry Mint Lemonade; 49

Red Cabbage and Cranberry Slaw; 45

Rice Cake with Almond Butter & Banana Slices; 46

Rice Pudding with Raisins and Cinnamon; 61

Salmon with Zesty Lemon Herb Drizzle; 35

Seasonal Fruit Salad with Fresh Mint; 70

Shrimp and Asparagus Stir-Fry; 37

Silky Chocolate Pudding; 55

Spinach and Mushroom Scramble; 20

Strawberry Sorbet; 56

Stuffed Bell Peppers with Ground Turkey; 41

Sunny Tuna Salad Sandwich; 24

Sunrise Berry Oatmeal; 16

Tofu and Snow Pea Stir-Fry; 36

Tofu Stir-Fry with Mixed Vegetables; 31

Tomato and Basil Scramble; 20

Turkey and Avocado Wrap; 30

Turkey and Mushroom Stew; 34

Turkey Meatballs with Marinara Sauce; 39

Veggie-Loaded Scrambled Eggs; 19

Vibrant Veggie Stir-Fry; 36

Zesty Lemon Tuna Salad Wrap; 25

Zesty Lemonade; 49

Thanks and see you next Book !

Joyna E. Dwait

Made in the USA
Las Vegas, NV
17 September 2024